Called to Give Life:

Second edition with discussion questions

a primer on the
Blessings of Children
and the
Harm of Contraception

Jason T. Adams

One More Soul
1846 N. Main Street
Dayton, Ohio 45405-3832
Phone: 1-800-307-7685
E-mail: omsoul@omsoul.com
www.OMSoul.com

Nihil Obstat

Rev. David L. Zink, Censor Deputatus

North Star, Ohio

January 31, 2003

Imprimatur

Most Rev. Carl K. Moeddel dec'd 2009
Former Vicar General and Auxiliary Bishop of Cincinnati

February 3, 2003

The *Nihil Obstat* and *Imprimatur* are a declaration that a book or pamphlet is considered to be free of doctrinal or moral error. It is not implied that those who have granted the *Nihil Obstat* or *Imprimatur* agree with the contents, opinions, or statements expressed.

Copyright © 2003, 2013

One More Soul

ISBN 0-9669777-6-9

A Publication of

One More Soul
1846 N. Main Street
Dayton, Ohio 45405-3832

Blessing

I pray that this sourcebook for catechesis will help many people understand the blessings that children bring and the value of human life. May ***Called to Give Life*** assist many people to understand ever more deeply the Church's teaching on marriage and contraception. May it be a great support to numerous families as they pursue their vocation of holiness and joyful fulfillment. May it reinforce in young people the ideals of Christian married love and the need to follow Christ's way of life.

With prayerful good wishes for the success of your efforts, I remain

Justin Rigali

Cardinal Justin Rigali
Former Archbishop of Philadelphia

Table of Contents

Abbreviations Key	vi
Acknowledgments	vii
Foreword	viii

Part I: Foundations — 1

Introduction	3
Chapter 1: Moral Considerations	7
Chapter 2: Biblical Considerations	23
Chapter 3: The Voice of the Fathers	33
Chapter 4: Modern Magisterial Teachings	43
Chapter 5: Natural Family Planning	53
Chapter 6: The Connection between Contraception and Abortion	63
Chapter 7: Authority and Dissent	69
Chapter 8: The Blessings of Children	77
Chapter 9: How should a couple discern "just" and "serious" reasons for postponing pregnancy?	83

Part II: Pastoral Considerations — 97

How faith communities can create an NFP culture liberated from contraception and open to the blessings of children	99
Opportunities for an NFP Homily	105
Conclusion	119
Preaching NFP: Why Not? Theresa Notare, Special Assistant of the Diocesan Development Program for Natural Family Planning (USCCB)	125
A Pastoral Letter on Marriage and the Family Most Reverend Harry J. Flynn	129

Appendix: Homilies (in alphabetical order by author) 135

   Homily Guide 137

   The Pill, the Pope, the Problem—Fr. Walter Austin 143

   Proclaiming Truth in and out of Season —Fr. John Bateman 147

   "Woman, How Great Is Your Faith!"—Fr. Phillip Bloom 152

   Seek and You Shall Find: The Beauty of Humanae Vitae—Fr. McLean Cummings 155

   Children Make Us More Human—Fr. Brian Doerr 158

   Revisiting Humanae Vitae—Most Reverend John F. Donoghue, DD 162

   God's Plan for Human Life—Fr. Matthew Habiger, OSB, PhD 166

   Trinity Sunday Homily—Fr. Matthew Habiger, OSB, PhD 170

   The Church's Moral Teaching on Contraception (a series of 3 sermons)
   —Fr. Anthony Kopp, O Praem

      (1) 23rd Sunday, Ordinary Time, Cycle A 173

      (2) 25th Sunday, Ordinary Time, Cycle A 178

      (3) Respect Life Sunday, 27th Sunday, Ordinary Time, Cycle A 182

   Anti-life Message Finds a Home in Contraception—Most Reverend Paul S. Loverde, DD, STL, JCL 188

   Love Means Giving Oneself Away—Most Reverend Thomas J. Olmstead 191

   Mass Commemorating the 30th Anniversary of Humanae Vitae—Justin Cardinal Rigali, JCD 195

Perceiving the Contraception Connection—Fr. Raymond Suriani 200

"This Sort of Talk Is Hard to Endure! How Can Anyone Take It Seriously?"—Fr. Joseph Taphorn 204

Additional Resources 207

What Is One More Soul? 213

About the Author 215

Abbreviations Key

AAS = *Acta Apostolicae Sedis* **(The Vatican Gazette, carries the original text of major Vatican documents)**

CCC = *The Catechism of the Catholic Church*

EV = *Evangelium Vitae (The Gospel of Life)*

FC = *Familiaris Consortio (On the Family)*

HV = *Humanae Vitae (Of Human Life)*

GS = *Gaudium et Spes (Pastoral Constitution on the Church in the Modern World)*

Acknowledgments

I would like to express my gratitude to the following people for their contributions:

Linda, my wife, for her encouragement and for her patience with the long hours it took to complete this project;

Steve Koob, director of *One More Soul*, for supporting *Called to Give Life* with his time, talent, and resources;

Vince Sacksteder, Resource Editor at *One More Soul*, for editorial, technical assistance, and comic relief;

Lisamarie Griffin, former outreach coordinator for *One More Soul*, for helping to collect and review homilies in the early stages of the project;

Sam & Beth Torode, authors of *Open Embrace*, for creating our original cover design at no charge;

Donna Griffin for her editorial input, and the rest of the staff at *One More Soul* who played a role in bringing this book to fruition;

Father Charles Mangan, whose article, "The Homily That Never Was" (*Homiletic and Pastoral Review*, November, 1991, pp. 67-70) has been a source of inspiration for the book.

***

Additionally, *One More Soul* would like to thank those who reviewed prepublication drafts of *Called to Give Life*, the many priests who contributed homilies for the book, and *One More Soul* benefactors who provide prayer and financial support for projects such as this. May God bless you all for your generosity.

Foreword

A great need exists not only in the Church but also in society for a return to authentic married and family life. Married men and women are called to a vocation of love—a vocation built on the universal call to holiness of all Christians.

Pope John Paul II in his Apostolic Letter, *Novo Millennio Ineunte*, calls us back to God's plan for married love. He stresses that, "...it is necessary to ensure that through an ever more complete Gospel formation, Christian families show convincingly that it is possible to live marriage fully in keeping with God's plan and with the true good of the human person..." (NMI 47). Jason Adams' book, *Called to Give Life: A Sourcebook on the Blessings of Children and the Harm of Contraception*, does just that.

Called to Give Life helps those who have the task of forming others to understand the wisdom of the Church's teachings about human sexuality. This sourcebook contains a bounty of information to help those in catechesis not only form others but also themselves. Part I provides vital documentation to explain the "whats and whys" behind the dangers of contraception, sterilization and abortion and the beauty of Natural Family Planning. Part II is a collection of homilies designed to help priests and deacons preach the truth of married love with courage. *Called to Give Life* concludes with an excellent section on pastoral considerations to make present and alive in dioceses and parishes the truth about human sexuality.

Jesus came that we may have life—and have it abundantly (cf. John 10:10). He calls married men and women to model His relationship to us, His Church. He earnestly desires married couples to bring forth new life through their loving relationships. Christian families must show the world that it is possible to live in keeping with the call of Christ. The Church has an obligation to call her sons and daughters to a life built on self-giving love. However, we cannot expect couples to live authentic married lives if we do not give them the tools with which to live. *Called to Give Life* is such a tool, and in the hands of dedicated parents, priests, deacons, and catechists we can help build a culture of life built on a civilization of love.

+Most Reverend Charles J. Chaput, O.F.M. Cap.
Archbishop of Philadelphia

This book is dedicated to my wife, Linda, whose example makes the ideal of self-sacrificial love—so central to God's plan for married life—real to me.

Part 1
Foundations

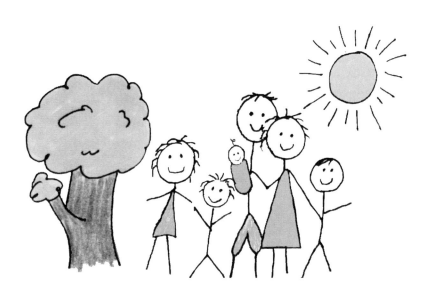

Introduction
Called to Give Life

"Called to give life, spouses share in the creative power and fatherhood of God" (CCC 2367). The transmission of human life is profoundly exemplary of the cooperation between God and humanity in the work of redemption. Since the dawn of creation God's children have been brought forth to share consciously in the very life of God, a dignity that is unique to the human species.

The means and the end of redemption are the sharing of God's life. When in marriage, a man and woman bring forth new life, they cooperate with God in the creation of a person with an immortal soul. This person, the integration of matter and spirit, is a sacramental being–a visible sign that shows forth an invisible reality. In this sense, the human person is an instrument of God's presence in the world, a walking, talking witness to God.

God's mysterious intervention in this process gives evidence that the new child, conceived of from eternity in the mind of God, is an integral part of God's plan: "Blessed be the God and Father of our Lord Jesus Christ, who has blessed us in Christ with every spiritual blessing in the heavenly places, even as he chose us in him before the foundation of the world, that we should be holy and blameless before him. He destined us in love to be his sons through Jesus Christ, according to the purpose of his will, to the praise of his glorious grace, which he freely bestowed on us in the Beloved" (Eph 1:3-6).

The marital act, in this light, becomes a co-creative act, willed by God through the love of spouses to produce a new and unique agent in salvation history. God's plan reaches the universal family of God through the individual family: "it must be said that true married love and the family life which flows from it have this end in view: that the spouses would cooperate generously with the love of the Creator and Savior, who through them will in due time increase and enrich His family" (GS 50). This is why God and his instrument of salvation on earth, the Church, take such great interest in the *means* by which we transmit human life. For underlying the procreation of children is the mission of the Church to redeem the world.

If you think this is overstating the case, you already underestimate the great power and purpose that lie within the marital act. In his infinite wisdom, God chose to make known his works and his inner life with the cooperation of human beings. He did this not because he needed us to achieve his plan for the universe, but because by co-creating with God we participate in his work of redemption: *our* dignity is heightened. When we procreate, we serve both of these ends; we provide the active instruments of salvation (new children of God) and in the process realize that thing that makes us most resemble God, our ability to bring forth life. Pope John Paul II describes this twofold end: "when…couples respect the inseparable connection between the unitive and procreative meanings of human sexuality, they are acting as 'ministers' of God's plan and they 'benefit from' their sexuality according to the original dynamism of 'total' self-giving" (FC 32).

It is with these ideals in sight that One More Soul brings you *Called to Give Life: A Sourcebook on the Blessings of Children and the Harm of Contraception*. The purpose of this book is to facilitate the work of pastoral ministers, catechists, and parents in matters of fertility: specifically, the blessings of children, Natural Family Planning, contraception, sterilization, in vitro fertilization, artificial reproductive technologies, and the providence of God in marital sexuality.

The book combines theory and practice, foundations and applications. It begins with the foundational concepts that drive fertility issues. Sources include Tradition and Scripture, Magisterial statements, theological reflections, considerations of the natural law, human experience, and recent statements from the bishops. Part I, *Foundations*, is a compilation of Biblical and theological rudiments–the essential rationale that undergirds the Church's vision of marital love and which drives the Church's shepherding of human fertility. Part II, *Pastoral Considerations*, is geared at implementation: that is, creating a family/parish/school culture free from contraception and open to the blessings of children. It includes an abundance of practical suggestions for creating the culture of life within a parish. The Appendix, *Homilies*, is a collection of homilies given by priests and bishops, compiled over the last several years. The purpose of making these homilies available is threefold: (1) to provide examples of homilies for clergy (bishops, priests, and deacons) interested in preaching on contraception, the blessings of children, and other fertility issues; (2) to provide encouragement to clergy that it *is* possible, indeed, *fruitful* to offer homilies on these issues; and (3) to provide the lay faithful access to homilies that they might not be getting in their parishes. Hence, the homilies section is not geared exclusively to the clergy; it is also geared to the laity for their spiritual enrichment and for their work in either adult catechesis or their universal calling to be ministers of truth in the workaday world. We at *One More Soul*, a national organization that exists for the purpose of making known the blessings of children and the harm of contraception, intend this book as a means of facilitating education in fertility issues for structured approaches–homilies, adult catechesis, marriage preparation, and RCIA–and also for the day to day conversation between families, friends, classmates, and coworkers that is perhaps just as influential.

To the cynical observer, it may seem that modern culture has fallen to the counterfeit freedom and shallow allurement of the *culture of death* and its "brave new world" of abortion, contraception, sterilization, and morbid control over the transmission of human life. The more hopeful outlook, as we see it, is a grassroots desire for and recovery of authentic freedom. While the contraceptive mentality binds us to the narrow confines of self-interest and *self-assertion*, openness to fertility extends our horizons and liberates us toward a life of unfettered generosity and *self-gift*. In this light, the issue of contraception is not viewed narrowly as one among many bioethical controversies, but as a window through which we view the interior life and our Savior's commandment, "Love one another as I love you" (John 15:12). Our personal fulfillment and our communal welfare depend on our ability to love one another. Contraception hinders our fulfillment as persons, and constitutes an obstacle to inner peace and happiness. It is our aim to remove this obstacle so that all of us can live joyfully and meaningfully.

Jason T. Adams
Author

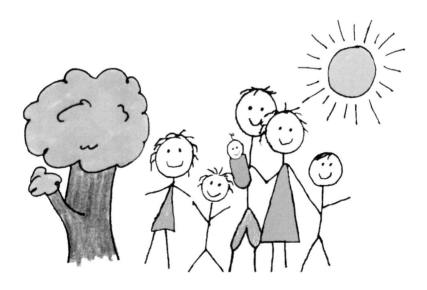

Chapter 1
Moral Considerations

"Any use whatsoever of matrimony exercised in such a way that the [sexual] act is deliberately frustrated in its natural power to generate life is an offense against the law of God and of nature, and those who indulge in such are branded with the guilt of grave sin."

   Pope Pius XI, *Casti Connubii 56*

Why is contraception immoral?

Too often the discussion of the morality of contraception fragments into a specific treatment of individual devices and methods wherein the overarching theological and philosophical essence of contraception is obfuscated. We lose sight of the forest for the trees. Behind every device and method of contraception is a fundamental breach of God's design for marital sexuality. Without this perspective, the Church's condemnation of contraception might appear to be a knee-jerk reaction to modernity or a rejection of science and man's dominion over the material universe. The more we can recover the root of the Church's prohibition of contraception, the more consistent and comprehensive will be our objections.

What is contraception?

In order to discuss the morality of a thing, we must first define it. *Contraception*, from the Latin *contra* (against) and *conceptio* (to conceive), literally means "against conception." It may be defined as "every action which, whether in anticipation of the conjugal act, or in its accomplishment, or in the development of its natural consequences, proposes, whether as an end or as a means, to render procreation impossible" (HV 14). Simply put, contraception is any intentional attempt to render the conjugal act infertile. Father Ronald Lawler and Dr. William May elaborate:

> Contraception, as the word itself suggests, is actively aimed at preventing conception. But it is necessary to begin with a clear definition of 'contraception' to make unmistakable the precise nature of the acts to which moral judgments about contraception are intended to apply.
>
> In his encyclical *Humanae Vitae*, Paul VI gave an exact account of the nature of contraceptive actions. A contraceptive act is had in any act of coition which is intended precisely to act against the procreative good, to prevent it from being realized…Thus, there are various ways in which intercourse can be contraceptive: through the use of mechanical devices (such as condoms or diaphragms), by the use of withdrawal or spermicides, by the use of anovulant pills, by surgical sterilization, and the like. Contraception is always part of a dual act, 'contraceptive intercourse.' In this dual act of contraceptive intercourse, one chooses to engage in sexual intercourse. While choosing to have intercourse, which is known to be essentially related to

the procreation of new human life, and precisely because one does not want the act of intercourse to flower the fruitfulness which it can have, one performs the contraceptive act. This act is aimed precisely against the procreative good. The coming-to-be of a new human life (which is in itself a great good, though one may perhaps very reasonably desire not to realize it here and now) is treated as an evil, something to be acted against. The precise purpose of the contraceptive act, as we shall more fully show below, is to act directly against the great human good of procreation–to treat it as if here and now it was an evil, not a good.

Contraception or contraceptive intercourse therefore is not identical in meaning with birth control or family planning. Plainly there are other ways to control births and to plan one's family than by engaging in contraceptive intercourse. One can control or prevent births by means far worse than contraception–by abortion, for instance. And one can plan one's family by means that are in themselves thoroughly good–that is, by Natural Family Planning.[1]

Note that in this definition contraception is not regarded as a classification of *things* alone that act against conception, but that it extends to the broader consideration of action, that is, a choice or act of the will against the natural fertility of sex. Hence it is not the material artificiality of contraception, the interference of *man-made* devices with a God-given faculty, alone that makes it unnatural. The artificiality of contraception extends to the willful frustration of one's true end. In other words, it violates the natural law, the purpose for which man and marriage were designed:

> Contrary to popular belief, the Church does not oppose artificial birth control *because* it's artificial. She opposes it because it's *contraceptive*. Contraception is the choice by any means *to impede the procreative potential of a given act of intercourse*. In other words, the contracepting couple chooses to engage in intercourse, and, foreseeing that their act may result in a new life, they *intentionally* and *willfully* suppress their fertility.[2]

A further point to be made is that, even if couples do not impede the procreative potential of a given act of intercourse, (i.e., even if they do not

---

[1] Lawler, Ronald, O.F.M., Cap., et al. *Catholic Sexual Ethics*. Our Sunday Visitor, Huntington, Indiana: 1996, pp.153-154.

[2] West, Christopher. *Good News About Sex & Marriage: Answers to Your Honest Questions about Catholic Teaching*. Charis/Servant Publications, Ann Arbor, Michigan: 2000, p.112.

contracept), they may well be engaging in their acts of intercourse with a mentality opposed to the good of children. Such a mentality (some call it a "contraceptive mentality") is utterly contrary to the meaning of marital love. It can develop even in a couple that practices natural means of birth regulation if the couple begins to see fertility as a disease to be avoided at all costs. While engaging in an act of intercourse with an anti-child mentality is not the moral equivalent of engaging in contracepted intercourse, it springs from the same disordered view of fertility and may result in a sort of rebellion against the goods of marriage.

In order to determine, therefore, what constitutes a violation of the procreative meaning of intercourse, we must not only ask what method is being used to regulate birth (means) but what is our intention, our motivation, our attitude toward the goods of marriage? In *Humanae Vitae* Pope Paul VI refers to the inseparability of the unitive and procreative meanings of intercourse. Since these two meanings of the act are truly inseparable, contraception wars against both. Contraception is a wholesale violation of the meaning of marital love. We have arrived, therefore, at an even broader understanding of the "contraceptive act": any act of intercourse that separates or opposes the procreative and unitive goods of marital sex.[3]

Why is contraception wrong?

❶ Contraception willfully divides the unitive and procreative aspects of sex.

That contraception deliberately separates the unitive and procreative aspects of sex is affirmed by John Paul II in his 1994 *Letter to Families*:

> In particular, responsible fatherhood and motherhood directly concern the moment in which a man and a woman, uniting themselves in one flesh, can become parents. This is a moment of special value both for their interpersonal relationship and for their service to life: They can become parents—father and mother—by communicating life to a new human being. The two dimensions of conjugal union, the unitive and the procreative, cannot be artificially separated without damaging the deepest truth of the conjugal act itself (12).

---

[3] Note that this discussion encompasses premarital sex. Fornication is a violation of the procreative aspect of marriage in that it denies the right of children to be born into a permanent union of mother and father (i.e., a family). It furthermore violates the unitive end of marriage insofar as "unitive" is understood to mean the permanent and unbreakable communion of persons that constitutes marriage.

(a) *Why are the unitive and procreative aspects of marital sex so important?*

Marriage, because it is part of God's plan to redeem and sanctify the world, has specific divinely instituted ends or goods. While secular culture may view marriage as a civil institution that is reducible to a contract, the concept of Christian marriage is founded on the mystery that marriage is a sacramental covenant communion in which two become one for the sake of their own salvation and the salvation of the world.

> The matrimonial covenant, by which a man and a woman establish between themselves a partnership of the whole of life, is by its nature ordered toward the good of the spouses and the procreation and education of offspring; this covenant between baptized persons has been raised by Christ the Lord to the dignity of a sacrament (CCC 1601).

A definition of the unitive and procreative elements of marriage will help demonstrate the salvific power of marriage and the indissoluble relationship between the unitive and procreative aspects of the marital act. The unitive aspect of marriage can be understood as the mutual and total self-giving of spouses to each other's salvation. The procreative aspect is the participation of the spouses in the creation of new life. The mutual commitment to salvation that characterizes the unitive aspect overflows to another person: the child. Love, by its nature grows; it never suppresses a good. Love is complete giving. Because it delights in the good of another, it is generous and unreserved.

The marital act is the visible sign of this overflowing of love. It visibly encapsulates the union between spouses and its life-giving power. Just as marriage integrates unitive and procreative, so must the physical expression of spousal communion. To separate the unitive from the procreative in the marital act is to disintegrate it and to frustrate God's plan for marriage.

Marriage is designed to give life, not to turn inward on itself. The grace of God that exists in the love of spouses is meant to overflow to the world. God gives life and love abundantly and expects us to do the same. This is why Christ established marriage as a sacrament that signifies His own fecund relationship with the Church:

> Husbands, love your wives, even as Christ loved the Church and handed himself over for her to sanctify her, cleansing her by the bath of water with the word, that he might present to himself the Church in splendor, without spot or wrinkle or any such thing, that she might be holy and without blemish. So also

husbands should love their wives as their own bodies. He who loves his wife loves himself. For no one hates his own flesh but rather nourishes and cherishes it, even as Christ does the Church, because we are members of his body.

> 'For this reason a man shall leave his father and his mother and be joined to his wife, and the two shall become one flesh.'

> This is a great mystery, but I speak in reference to Christ and the Church. In any case, each one of you should love his wife as himself, and the wife should respect her husband (Eph 5:25-33).

Christ espouses His Church, our mother, and in this covenant there is a mutual outpouring of self in which nothing is held back, even to the point of giving one's own life. The communion that exists between Christ and His Bride brings forth new life—spiritual children who deepen the life of the Church. In the same way, marriage must be life-giving. Spouses must exhibit the same total self-gift that Christ offered, holding nothing back—including their fertility. Christ's love for His Church is never contraceptive, never self-gratifying, but exists for the very purpose of creating new life.

Consider an entity in which two people love each other so much that they exist as one, and in which the love of this union is so real and so intense that another person proceeds from it, a person who is sent out into the world to sanctify it. Sound familiar? The life-giving love of family is analogous to the inner life of God himself. Pope John Paul II writes: "God in his deepest mystery is not a solitude, but a family, since He has in Himself fatherhood, sonship, and the essence of the family which is love."[4] When we live according to this mystery we conform to the image of God; when we live counter to it we deviate from the image of God.

As a communion of persons, the marriage that is open to children witnesses to the world the very life of God:

> The Christian family is a communion of persons, a sign and image of the communion of the Father and the Son in the Holy Spirit. In the procreation and education of children it reflects the Father's work of creation. It is called to partake of the prayer and sacrifice of Christ...The Christian family has an evangelizing and missionary task (CCC 2205).

---

[4] in Hahn, Scott, *A Father Who Keeps His Promises,* Charis (Servant), Ann Arbor, MI, 1998, p. 36.

This is the exalted dignity of marriage, expressed by the cooperation of unitive and procreative elements. To deny either is to deny the divine calling that makes marriage part of God's plan.

> (b) Isn't this philosophical hair-splitting? Does God really delineate marital sex into its unitive and procreative aspects?

If it seems unlikely that God would engage in categorizing and defining the aspects of marital sex, it is only because we know that God sees things in wholes, not in parts. God gets to the essence of things and so should we. This is why the Church exhorts her children to observe sex in its wholeness, not separating unitive and procreative. Parsing sex into categories comes about as a response to our abuse of its integrity.

Catechism Connection

The Unitive and Procreative Ends of the Marital Embrace

The spouses' union achieves the twofold end of marriage: the good of the spouses themselves and the transmission of life. These two meanings or values of marriage cannot be separated without altering the couple's spiritual life and compromising the goods of marriage and the future of the family. The conjugal love of man and woman thus stands under the twofold obligation of fidelity and fecundity (2363).

Fecundity is a gift, and *end of marriage*, for conjugal love naturally tends to be fruitful. A child does not come from outside as something added on to the mutual love of the spouses, but springs from the very heart of that mutual giving as its fruit and fulfillment. So the Church, which 'is on the side of life' teaches that 'each and every marriage act must remain open to the transmission of life.' 'This particular doctrine, expounded on numerous occasions by the Magisterium, is based on the inseparable connection, established by God, which man on his own initiative may not break, between the unitive significance and the procreative significance which are both inherent to the marriage act (CCC 2366).

---

❷ The practice of contraception holds that man, apart from God, is the overseer of when life shall begin.

Pope John Paul II explains:

> At the origin of every human person there is a creative act of God… [I]t follows that the procreative capacity, inscribed in

human sexuality, is—in its deepest truth—a cooperation with God's creative power. It also follows that men and women are not the arbiters, are not the masters of this same capacity, called as they are, in it and through it, to be participants in God's creative decision. When, therefore, through contraception, married couples remove from the exercise of their conjugal sexuality its potential procreative capacity, they claim a power which belongs solely to God: the power to decide, in *a final analysis*, the coming into existence of a human person. They assume the qualification not of being cooperators in God's creative power, but the ultimate depositories of the source of human life… [C]ontraception is…so profoundly unlawful as never to be, for any reason, justified. To think or to say the contrary is equal to maintaining that in human life situations may arise in which it is lawful not to recognize God as God.[5]

This, according to Dietrich Von Hildebrand, is the sin of irreverence:

> The sinfulness of birth control is rooted in the arrogation of the right to separate the actualized love union in marriage from a possible conception, to sever the wonderful, deeply mysterious connection instituted by God. This mystery is approached in an irreverent attitude. We are here confronted with the fundamental sin of irreverence toward God, the denial of our creaturehood, the acting as if we were our own lords. This is a basic denial of our being bound to God: it is a disrespect for the mysteries of God's creation, and its sinfulness increases with the rank of the mystery in question. It is the same sinfulness that lies in suicide or in euthanasia, in both of which we act as if we were masters of life.
>
> Every *active* intervention of the spouses that eliminates the possibility of conception through the conjugal act is incompatible with the holy mystery of the superabundant relation in this incredible gift of God. And this irreverence also affects the purity of the conjugal act, because the union can be the real fulfillment of love only when it is approached with reverence and when it is embedded in the consciousness of our basic bond to God…
>
> We thus see that artificial birth control is sinful not only because it severs the mysterious link between the most intimate love union and the coming into existence of a new human being, but also because in a certain way it artificially cuts off the creative intervention of God, or better still, it artificially separates an act which is ordained toward cooperation with the creative act of God

---

[5] Pope John Paul II, Discourse, Sept. 17, 1983; 28 *The Pope Speaks* 356, 356-57 (1983); as quoted in *The Winning Side*, Dr. Charles Rice, p.109.

from this, its destiny. For, as Paul VI says, this is to consider oneself not a servant of God, but "Lord over the origin of human life."[6]

❸ Contraception impairs the full reciprocal self-offering that constitutes the marital embrace.

In his 1981 Apostolic Exhortation *Familiaris Consortio*, Pope John Paul II describes this reservation of self in the marital embrace as an "objectively contradictory language":

> When couples, by means of recourse to contraception, separate these two meanings that God the Creator has inscribed in the being of man and woman and in the dynamism of their sexual communion, they act as "arbiters" of the divine plan and they "manipulate" and degrade human sexuality and with it themselves and their married partner by altering its value of "total" self-giving. Thus the innate language that expresses the total reciprocal self-giving of husband and wife is overlaid through contraception, by an objectively contradictory language, namely, that of not giving oneself totally to the other. This leads not only to a positive refusal to be open to life but also to a falsification of the inner truth of conjugal love, which is called upon to give itself in personal totality (32).

The Most Reverend John J. Meyers, Archbishop of Newark, explains the Holy Father's formulation:[7]

> John Paul II roots the entire Christian sexual ethic not only in the *structure of the act* (though he acknowledges its importance), but rather in the meaning of the love reflected in sexual intercourse. Couples readily assent to the teaching that the *normal* meaning of intercourse is mutual love. They can also readily assent to the teaching that the *ultimate* meaning of sexual intercourse is when their love for each other can produce new life, if it be God's will.
>
> What they are *gradually* beginning to see is that within this context, it is morally dishonest to withhold part of that love through contraceptive intercourse.
>
> Long before he became Pope, John Paul taught at length on sexual morality. He maintained that the only proper response to

---

[6] Von Hildebrand, Dietrich. *Love, Marriage, and the Catholic Conscience: Understanding the Church's Teachings on Birth Control*. Sophia Institute Press, Manchester, New Hampshire: 1998, pp.45-46.

[7] The following is excerpted from Bishop John J Meyers, "The Rejection and Rediscovery by Christians of the Truths of Humanae Vitae," *Trust the Truth*, The Pope John Center, Braintree, Massachusetts: 1991.

a person is *love*. For him, a person could never be reduced to the level of an *object*, a means to an end. Contraceptive intercourse, he posited, is one way in which married couples sin against one another, their own love, and the Creator, by reducing the other to a means of pleasure.

Moreover, as Pope, John Paul II has explored the marriage relationship more deeply. He has repeatedly explored the "language of the body." The human body, with its sexual dimension seen in the very mystery of creation, is not only a source of fruitfulness and procreation, as in the whole natural order, but includes right from the beginning the "nuptial" attribute, that is, the capacity for expressing love—that love precisely in which the man-person becomes a gift, and by means of that gift, fulfills the very meaning of his being and existence.[8]

The conjugal act is 'true' only when the conjugal love which it expresses is true. As the Holy Father states: "In the act which expresses their conjugal love, the spouses are called to make *of themselves* a gift, one to the other: nothing of what constitutes their *being* a person may be excluded from this self donation."[9]

Contraception introduces a limitation on the self-giving of the other, and therefore a falsification which contradicts true married love.

Married couples are *gradually* beginning to see the core *practical* teaching of the Holy Father: that married couples may engage in conjugal relations whenever they wish, but they must *mean what they are saying with their bodies.*

Pope John Paul II has, in other words, fueled a reexamination of the Church's teaching on fertility and contraception by expanding the Church's definition of contraception from the unlawful and unnatural sterilization of the sexual act, to the deeper and more comprehensive sterilization of *human love* and mutual self-gift:

> Man and woman carry on in the language of the body that dialogue which, according to Genesis 2:24, 25, had its beginning on the day of creation. This language of the body is something more than mere sexual reaction. As authentic language of the persons, it is subject to the demands of truth, that is, to objective moral norms. Precisely on the level of this language, man and woman reciprocally express themselves in the fullest and most profound way possible to them by the corporeal dimension of masculinity and femininity. Man and woman express themselves in the measure of the whole truth of the human person.

---

[8] John Paul II, General Audience, 16 January, 1980.
[9] John Paul II, *Discourse on Responsible Parenthood*, 17 September, 1983.

Man is precisely a person because he is master of himself and has self-control. Indeed, insofar as he is master of himself he can give himself to the other. This dimension—the dimension of the liberty of the gift—becomes essential and decisive for that language of the body, in which man and woman reciprocally express themselves in the conjugal union. Granted that this is communion of persons, the language of the body should be judged according to this criterion of truth...

According to the criterion of this truth, which should be expressed in the language of the body, the conjugal act signifies not only love, but also potential fecundity. Therefore it cannot be deprived of its full and adequate significance by artificial means. In the conjugal act it is not licit to separate the unitive aspect from the procreative aspect, because both the one and the other pertain to the intimate truth of the conjugal act. The one is activated together with the other and in a certain sense the one by means of the other... Therefore, in such a case the conjugal act, deprived of its interior truth because it is artificially deprived of its procreative capacity, ceases also to be an act of love.

It can be said that in the case of an artificial separation of these two aspects, a real bodily union is carried out in the conjugal act, but it does not correspond to the interior truth and to the dignity of personal communion—communion of persons. This communion demands that the language of the body be expressed reciprocally in the integral truth of its meaning. If this truth be lacking, one cannot speak either of the truth of self-mastery, or of the truth of the reciprocal gift and of the reciprocal acceptance of self on the part of the person. Such a violation of the interior constitutes the essential evil of the contraceptive act.[10]

In their expression of marital sexuality, the couple signifies bodily such mutual, self-emptying love as Christ Himself poured forth on the Cross. For this reason, some in the Church have referred to the Crucifixion as the consummation of the union between Christ, the Bridegroom, and his bride, the Church. To deprive the marital act of its mutually self-emptying capacity by withholding one's generative power, is, simply put, a lie. One "speaks" with one's body what one does not mean interiorly. A communion of persons, which is the rightful end of the sexual act, cannot be achieved with such a reservation. Contraception is a violation of the communion for which sexuality is directed in the first place.

---

[10] General Audience, August 22, 1984.

Bishops Speak

Most Reverend Charles J. Chaput, OFM Cap, Archbishop of Philadelphia

The covenant which husband and wife enter at marriage requires that *all* intercourse remain open to the transmission of new life. This is what becoming "one flesh" implies: complete self-giving, without reservation or exception, just as Christ withheld nothing of Himself from His bride, the Church, by dying for her on the cross. *Any* intentional interference with the procreative nature of intercourse necessarily involves spouses' withholding themselves from each other and from God, who is their partner in sacramental love. In effect, they steal something infinitely precious—themselves—from each other and from their Creator.

Of Human Life: A Pastoral Letter to the People of God of Northern Colorado on the Truth and Meaning of Married Love: July 22, 1998.

Most Reverend Glennon P. Flavin, DD, Bishop Emeritus of Lincoln, Nebraska

Therefore, we who have been blessed by God with the gift of the Catholic Faith can have no doubt about the immorality of artificial contraception. The Catholic Church clearly teaches that the use of artificial contraception in all its forms, including direct sterilization, is gravely immoral, is intrinsically evil, is contrary to the law of nature and nature's God. This is and always has been the uninterrupted teaching of the Catholic Church from the beginning.

The ban on contraception is not a disciplinary law of the Church, like abstinence on Friday, which the Church can enact and which the Church can change and from which the Church can dispense for good reasons. Rather, it is a Divine Law which the Church cannot change any more than it can change the Law of God forbidding murder. Artificial contraception is wrong, not because the Church says it is wrong (it was wrong before Christ established the Church); it is wrong because God Himself, through the revelation of His Son, Our Lord Jesus Christ, has declared it to be wrong. Because artificial contraception is intrinsically evil, it may never be practiced for any reason, no matter how good and urgent. A good end never justifies the use of an evil means.

A Pastoral Letter to Catholic Couples and Physicians on the issue of Artificial Contraception: October 11, 1991.

> ## Did you know ...
> ### Catholics out-contracept the general population
> According to the 1995 National Survey of Family Growth, conducted by the National Center for Health Statistics, the percentage of Catholic women (ages 15-44) who were using some form of contraception was 70% versus a 64 % rate for women in the general population.
>
> In 1988, the most common form of contraception among Catholic women was oral contraception (the Pill). Whereas in the 1995 study, the most frequent form of contraception was sterilization. 40% of Catholic respondents reported the use of sterilization—that represents 4.8 million Catholic women ages 15-44. The rate of sterilization among Catholics doubled from 1988 to 1995.
>
> Only about 3% of Catholic women using a method of birth regulation use Natural Family Planning: about 300-400 thousand women.
> *Richard J. Fehring, DNSc, RN, and Andrea Matovina Schlidt, BSN, RN. "Trends in Contraceptive Use Among Catholics in the United States." Linacre Quarterly, 68 (2): 170-185.*

Review Questions

1. How is contraception defined?

2. What are the various kinds of contraception?

3. What makes contraception unnatural?

4. What is the so-called "contraceptive mentality"? How would we know if we had a contraceptive mentality?

5. How is the "unitive" aspect of sex defined?

6. How is the "procreative" aspect of sex defined?

7. How does openness to children witness the life of God to the world?

8. How is contraception a "sterilization of human love and mutual self-gift"?

Discussion (Answers will vary)

1. Is the definition of contraception given here different from your prior/current understanding of contraception? If so, how?

2. Do you think contraception is commonly defined this way? What common definitions have you encountered?

3. What aspect(s) of the definition of contraception do you think are most misunderstood? Explain.

4. That the unitive and procreative aspects of sex cannot be separated implies their cooperation. How would you describe the interrelation of the two?

5. Why is it important that God is the overseer of when life begins?

6. Do you agree with Bishop John Meyer's statement (p.14): "Married couples are *gradually* beginning to see the core *practical* teaching of the Holy Father: that married couples may engage in conjugal relations whenever they wish, but they must *mean what they are saying with their bodies*"? How can we witness this principal to married couples to ensure that Bishop Meyer's claim is fully realized?

Materials in this book may be copied freely, without alteration, for non-commercial purposes.

Chapter 2
Biblical Considerations

"Be fertile and multiply; fill the earth and subdue it."

Genesis 1:28

What does the Bible say about contraception?

The Second Vatican Council's statement on Divine Revelation teaches us that interpretation of the Sacred Scriptures must devote attention to "the content and unity of the whole of scripture, taking into account the tradition of the entire Church…"[11] Much more than a moral manual or a doctrinal concordance, the Bible is an inspired expression of the faith and life of the Church. In contrast to the legalism of the Pharisees, the revelation of Christ was/is comprehensive, describing the positive fulfillment of the demands of love. Our application of this revelation to the specific moral questions of our age, in this case contraception, involves submitting our actions to the standard of life-giving love established by God, both in his fathering of the chosen people of old, and in his redemption of the New Israel.

The morality of contraception must be viewed in this light, that is, in the light of God's ineffable love for human life and his plan for its transmission. Looking to the Bible for guidance on the issue of contraception must consider the Bible's revelation of the sovereignty of God over creation and His plan for marriage. It must also recognize that Scripture reveals children as the supreme gift of marriage and a blessing from God.

---

❶ Subverting the sovereignty of God: the deliberate act of rendering a sexual act infertile.

▶ Genesis 38:8-10

The Bible contains teachings relevant to contraception on a variety of levels. The most direct of these references is Genesis 38:8-10, the *Onan Incident*:

> Then Judah said to Onan, "Go in to your brother's wife, and perform your duty as a brother-in-law to her, and raise up offspring for your brother." And Onan knew that the offspring would not be his; so it came about that when he went in to his brother's wife, he wasted his seed on the ground, in order not to give offspring to his brother. But what he did was displeasing in the sight of the Lord, so He took his life also.

Though God was certainly displeased with Onan's disobedience to the Levirate Law: that is, the obligation of a man to sow children with his dead brother's widow, his punishment for Onan far exceeded the penalty mandated for such a crime. According to Deuteronomy 25:5-10, the penalty

---

[11] *Dei Verbum*, no.12.

is for the slighted widow to publicly humiliate the offender. God's enactment of the death penalty for Onan indicates a heightened seriousness in the offense. The only additional element to Onan's refusal to provide offspring is his choice to make the sexual act deliberately infertile by withdrawal.

That Onan's punishment was due to his use of contraception is pointed out by Pope Pius XI in his encyclical *Casti Connubii*:

> Small wonder, therefore, if Holy Writ bears witness that the Divine Majesty regards with greatest detestation this horrible crime [contraception] and at times has punished it with death. As St. Augustine notes, 'Intercourse even with one's legitimate wife is unlawful and wicked where the conception of the offspring is prevented. Onan, the son of Judah, did this and the Lord killed him for it' (55).

Even the most notable Protestant theologians agree on this point. Martin Luther, for example, equates Onan's action with sodomy:

> Onan must have been a malicious and incorrigible scoundrel. This is a most disgraceful sin…We call it unchastity, yes, a Sodomitic sin. For Onan goes in to her; that is, he lies with her and copulates, and when it comes to the point of insemination, spills the semen, lest the woman conceive. Surely at such a time the order of nature established by God in procreation should be followed (Commentary on Genesis 38:8-10).[12]

Likewise, John Calvin, founder of Calvinism and other sects of Calvinist extraction such as Presbyterians and the United Church of Christ, calls Onan's withdrawal "monstrous":

> Besides, he [Onan] not only defrauded his brother of the right due him, but also preferred his semen to putrify on the ground, rather than to beget a son in his brother's name…The voluntary spilling of semen outside intercourse between man and woman is a monstrous thing. Deliberately to withdraw from coitus in order that semen may fall on the ground is doubly monstrous (Commentary on Genesis 38:8-10).[13]

❷ **Offspring are the supreme gift of marriage, a blessing from God through which God is revealed to the world.**

---

[12] Provan, Charles D. *The Bible and Birth Control*. Zimmer Printing. Monongahela, Pennsylvania: 1989, p.81.

The Image and Likeness of God

▶ **Genesis 1:27-28** (Easter Vigil; Tues Wk 5 Yr 1; Marriage)

"God created man in his image, in the divine image he created him; male and female he created them. God blessed them, saying: 'Be fruitful and multiply; fill the earth and subdue it.'"

▶ **Genesis 9:1** (Thurs Wk 6 Yr 1)

"God blessed Noah and his sons and said to them: 'Be fertile and multiply and fill the earth.'"

Guadium et Spes, the Second Vatican Council's *Pastoral Constitution on the Church in the Modern World*, discusses God's primordial plan for marriage and its natural openness to fertility:

> Children are the supreme gift of marriage and contribute greatly to the good of the parents themselves. God himself said: 'It is not good that man should be alone,' and 'from the beginning [he] made them male and female'; wishing to associate them in a special way in his own creative work, God blessed man and woman with the words: 'Be fruitful and multiply.' Hence, true married love and the whole structure of family life which results from it, without diminishment of the other ends of marriage, are directed to disposing the spouses to cooperate valiantly with the love of the Creator and Savior, who through them will increase and enrich his family from day to day (no. 50).

Endowed with the gift and responsibility to participate in God's redemption of humanity, the married couple perpetuates and projects the image and likeness of God in its transmission of life. In his explanation of the vows of Catholic marriage and the question as to whether the new couple will accept children from the Lord, Pope John Paul II teaches: "When the Church asks 'Are you willing?' she is reminding the bride and groom that they stand *before* the creative power of God. They are called to become parents, to cooperate with the Creator in giving life. Cooperating with God to call new human beings into existence means contributing to the transmission of that divine image and likeness of which everyone 'born of a woman' is a bearer."[14]

---

[13] Ibid., p.67.
[14] *Letter to Families from Pope John Paul II*, no.8.

> The procreation of children is a further revelation of the image and likeness of God in that it creates a communion of persons, a family, which signifies the communion of persons essential to Christ. "The Christian family is a communion of persons, a sign and image of the communion of the Father and the Son in the Holy Spirit. In the procreation and education of children it reflects the Father's work of creation" (CCC 2205).

▶ Malachi 2:14-15

"…the Lord is witness between you and the wife of your youth, with whom you have broken faith though she is your companion, your betrothed wife. Did he not make one being, with flesh and spirit: *and what does that one require but godly offspring?*"

While this verse occurs in the context of a discourse on the infidelity of God's people to the covenant wherein idolatry is likened to adultery, the point still holds. The analogy would make no sense if offspring were not customarily considered a necessary good of marriage. In other words, it is clear that offspring were considered the natural sign of a one-flesh union.

▶ 1 Timothy 2:15

"She will be saved through childbearing, provided she continues in faith and love and holiness—her chastity being taken for granted."

Here Paul proclaims the great dignity of the vocation of motherhood and its indispensable role in the plan of God for the salvation of parents. St. Paul, moreover, implies that the whole body of Christ benefits from cherishing the transmission of human life; for when a mother cooperates with God in the creation of new life and its Christian formation, she contributes to the building up of the Christian community. By definition, a vocation is a pathway of holiness that exists to fortify the Kingdom of God. Childbearing, depicted by Paul as a vocation, is no exception.

Catechism Connection: Children Are a Blessing from God

"Sacred Scripture and the Church's traditional practice see in large families a sign of God's blessing and the parents' generosity."
Catechism of the Catholic Church, 2373

▶ **Psalm 127:3-5**

"Behold sons are a gift from the Lord; the fruit of the womb is a reward. Like arrows in the hand of a warrior are the sons of one's youth. Happy the man whose quiver is filled with them; they shall not be put to shame when they contend with the enemies at the gate."

▶ **Psalm 128:1-4** (Holy Family; 27th Sunday B; 33d Sunday A; Thurs Wk 5 Yr 1; Thurs Wk 9 Yr 1; Fri Wk 12 Yr 1; Sat Wk 20 Yr 1; Wed Wk 21 Yr 2; Tues Wk 30 Yr 2; Common of Saints; Marriage)

"Happy are those who fear the Lord, who walk in his ways! For you shall eat the fruit of your handiwork; happy shall you be, and favored. Your wife shall be like a fruitful vine in the recesses of your home; your children like olive plants around your table. Behold, thus is the man blessed who fears the Lord."

▶ **Exodus 23:25-26**

"The Lord, your God, you shall worship; then I will bless your food and drink, and I will remove all sickness from your midst; *no woman in your land will be barren or miscarry*; and I will give you a full span of life."

▶ **Deuteronomy 7:13-14**

"As your reward for heeding these decrees and observing them carefully, the Lord, your God, will keep with you the merciful covenant which he promised on oath to your fathers. He will love and bless and multiply you; he will bless the fruit of your womb…. You will be blessed above all peoples; no man or woman among you shall be childless…."

Not only do these passages portray children as a natural blessing but as a transcendent blessing for fidelity to the covenant. As such, they are the *best* of what God offers for they are not just the natural reward of a well-ordered life but a divine premium that comes from the inner life of God. Before we receive them, they exist in the mind of God, worthy of his forethought and of his love. The Psalmist says, "*Truly you have formed my inmost being; you knit me in my mother's womb*" (Ps 139:13). How could we view children as anything but precious gifts into which God pours his very being—gifts that come from His heart to be received with awe and gratitude?

For this reason "Sacred Scripture and the Church's traditional practice see in *large families* a sign of God's blessing and the parents' generosity"(CCC 2373). Vatican II likewise teaches, "Among the married couples who thus fulfill their God-given mission, special mention should be made of those who after prudent reflection and joint decision courageously undertake the rearing of a large family" (GS 50).

▶ Pharmakos and pharmakeia in the New Testament (Gal. 5: 19-26, Rev. 9:21, Rev. 21:8)

Some scholars (cf Kimberly Hahn in *Life-Giving Love* [5]) hold that these New Testament words represent, in context, a stinging condemnation of contraception and chemical abortion. Usually translated as "sorcerer" and "sorcery," they refer more specifically to a mixer of potions or to the potions themselves, medicines that were commonly directed at preventing fertility or at achieving abortion.

> "Now the works of the flesh are obvious: immorality, impurity, licentiousness, idolatry, **sorcery**, hatreds…those who do such things will not inherit the kingdom of God." Gal. 5:19-20

> "Nor did they repent of their murders, their **magic potions**, their unchastity, or their robberies." Rev 9:21

> "But as for cowards, the unfaithful, the depraved, murderers, the unchaste, **sorcerers**, idol-worshipers, and deceivers of every sort, their lot is in the burning pool of fire and sulfur, which is the second death." Rev. 21:8

Summary

Putting the whole picture together, we start with God's "first commandment" to "increase and multiply," we browse through the Old Testament in which children are seen as some of the best blessings of God and even as a requirement for His people, and we finish with contraceptive practices being classed with "immorality, impurity, licentiousness, and idolatry" and also with "murders, unchastity, and robberies."

As we try to put on the heart of God, as revealed in the Scriptures, one of the main themes we encounter is His overflowing love for human life and especially for children. The fierce condemnation of immorality and of contraception in particular appear to reflect God's great desire that people enjoy the full joys and healing that come from loving family life and service to children.

What to do?

All of us are closely connected to people involved with contraception and many of us have used contraceptives or are still doing so. Many of us have been sterilized—the ultimate contraceptive. Knowing now how God approaches these matters, we have a great opportunity to help others to deeper life and to walk this way ourselves.

We are well aware of our weaknesses and others' as well. The full, abundant life of God, however, is waiting for us and for those we love, provided we open ourselves to it. One important step is simply to talk about the situation, to God, to each other, to a confessor, to a godly friend. If additional information is needed, One More Soul[6] has a wide range of teaching materials that can help, as well as recorded testimonies of couples who have struggled with this situation before. There are more people every day who have faced this crisis and come out healed. The possibilities are broad and full of hope.

Review Questions

1. How is Onan's death not just a punishment for not observing the Levirate law but a punishment for a contraceptive act?

2. Which passages of Scripture contain the divine mandate to procreate?

3. How is procreation a revelation of the image and likeness of God?

4. Does the New Testament say anything about contraception?

Discussion Questions

1. Why do you think God chose to perpetuate creation through the marital embrace, making us co-creators with him? In other words, what do you think is the purpose of this cooperation in God's plan?

2. The popular expression, "What would Jesus do?" reminds us that the moral life consists in conforming our lives to Christ. This being the case, what do we learn from Christ about the value of children? Use specific examples from Scripture.

Chapter 3
The Voice of the Fathers

"They [certain Egyptian heretics] exercise genital acts, yet prevent the conceiving of children. Not in order to produce offspring, but to satisfy lust, are they eager for corruption."

Epiphanius of Salamis:
Medicine Chest Against Heresies
26:5:2, AD 375

What does Tradition teach about contraception?

"Anthropological studies show that contraception is a social practice of much greater antiquity and cultural universality than was commonly supposed by medical and social historians. Medical papyri describing contraceptive methods are extant from 2700 BC in China, and from 1850 BC in Egypt."[15] Contraception is not a new phenomenon, and neither is the Church's condemnation of it. From the earliest teachings of the Church, contraception has been treated as a disordering of the goods of marriage and a threat to the spiritual welfare of its practitioners.

The statements that follow illustrate the continuity of the Church's teaching against contraception but, conditioned by the time in which they were written and the literary context in which they were treated, some are more denunciatory in tone than more contemporary expressions. Statements that associate the use of contraception with harlotry and homicide—for example, those of Chrysostom, Jerome, Augustine, and Caesarius of Arles—are given to hyperbole. While their expression is less "pastoral" than we are used to, they contain important truths about the grave disorderedness of contraceptive acts, and demonstrate the permanence of the Church's objection to the use of contraception.

▶ The Didache

> The Didache, or "The Teaching of the Twelve Apostles," composed near the end of the first century or the beginning of the second, was an early manual of Christian instruction.
>
> "You shall not use magic. You shall not use drugs. You shall not procure abortion. You shall not destroy a newborn child" (II, 2).
>
> In his *The Catholic Catechism*, father John Hardon S.J. explains this ancient prohibition:
>
>> Records from the practices of those times tell us that the people would first try some magical rites or resort to sorcery to avoid conception. If this failed, they would use one or another of the medical contraceptives elaborately described by Soranos [Ephesian gynecologist AD 98-138]. If notwithstanding a woman became pregnant, she would try to abort. And if even this failed, there was always the Roman law that permitted infanticide.[16]

---

[15] Hardon, John A., S.J. *The Catholic Catechism: A Contemporary Catechism of the Teachings of the Catholic Church*, Image Books/Doubleday, New York: 1981, p.367.
[16] Ibid., 367-368.

▶ **The Letter of Barnabas** *A late first, early second century epistle popular in the ancient Church. It was quoted by such Church Fathers as Clement of Alexandria and Origen.*

> [On the contraceptive character of orally consummated sex] "Moreover, he [Moses] has rightly detested the weasel [Lev. 11:29]. For he means, 'Thou shall not be like to those whom we hear of as committing wickedness with the mouth with the body through uncleanness [orally consummated sex]; nor shall thou be joined to those impure women who commit iniquity with the mouth with the body through uncleanness'" (*Letter of Barnabas* 10:8 [AD 74]).[17]

▶ **Clement of Alexandria** *Early Greek theologian; head of the catechetical school of Alexandria; d. 215.*

> "Because of its divine institution for the propagation of man, the seed is not to be vainly ejaculated, nor is it to be damaged, nor is it to be wasted" (*The Instructor of Children* 2:10:91:2 [AD 191]).

> "To have coitus other than to procreate children is to do injury to nature" (ibid., 2:10:95:3).

▶ **Hippolytus** *Martyr and presbyter; d. about 236.*

> [On Christian women with male concubines] "On account of their prominent ancestry and great property, the so-called faithful want no children from slaves or lowborn commoners, they use drugs of sterility [oral contraceptives] or bind themselves tightly in order to expel a fetus which has already been engendered [abortion]" (*Refutation of All Heresies* 9:12 [AD 225]).

▶ **Lactantius** *A Christian apologist of the fourth century.*

> "[Some] complain of the scantiness of their means, and allege that they have not enough for bringing up more children, as though, in truth, their means were in [their] power…or God did not daily make the rich poor and the poor rich. Wherefore, if any one on any account of poverty shall be unable to bring up children, it is better to abstain from relations with his wife" (*Divine Institutes* 6:20 [AD 307]).

> "God gave us eyes not to see and desire pleasure, but to see acts to be performed for the needs of life; so too, the genital ['generating'] part

---

[17] This and the following references are based on *Fathers Know Best: Contraception & Sterilization*, Catholic Answers, Inc., 1996; www.catholic.com/library/Contraception_and_Sterilization.asp.

of the body, as the name itself teaches, has been received by us for no other purpose than the generation of offspring" (ibid., 6:23:18).

▶ Council of Nicaea I *First ecumenical council of the Church*

[On the self-mutilative character of sterilization] "[I]f anyone in sound health has castrated [sterilized] himself, it behooves that such a one, if enrolled among the clergy, should cease [from his ministry], and that from henceforth no such person should be promoted. But, as it is evident that this is said of those who willfully do the thing and presume to castrate themselves, so if any have been made eunuchs by barbarians, or by their masters, and should otherwise be found worthy, such men this canon admits to the clergy" (canon 1 [AD 325]).

▶ Epiphanius of Salamis *Fourth century monk and bishop of Salamis (Constantia).*

"They [certain Egyptian heretics] exercise genital acts, yet prevent the conceiving of children. Not in order to produce offspring, but to satisfy lust, are they eager for corruption" (*Medicine Chest Against Heresies* 26:5:2 [AD 375]).

▶ John Chrysostom *Highly prominent doctor of the Greek Church; d. 407.*

[Contraception is likened to treated one's spouse as a prostitute] "Why do you sow where the field is eager to destroy the fruit, where there are medicines of sterility [oral contraceptives], where there is murder before birth? You do not even let a harlot remain only a harlot, but you make her a murderess as well…Indeed, it is something worse than murder, and I do not know what to call it; for she does not kill what is formed but prevents its formation. What then? Do you condemn the gift of God and fight with his [natural] laws?… [T]he matter still seems indifferent to many men—even to many men having wives. In this indifference of the married men there is greater evil filth; for then poisons are prepared, not against the womb of a prostitute, but against your injured wife. Against her are these innumerable tricks" (*Homilies on Romans* 24 [AD 391]).

"[I]n truth, all men know that they who are under the power of this disease [the sin of covetousness] are wearied even of their father's old age [wishing him to die so they can inherit]; and that which is sweet, and universally desirable, the having of children, they esteem grievous and unwelcome. Many at least with this view have even paid money to be childless, and have mutilated nature, not only killing the newborn, but even acting to prevent their beginning to live [sterilization]" (*Homilies on Matthew* 28:5 [AD 391]).

"[T]he man who has mutilated [sterilized] himself, in fact, is subject even to a curse, as Paul says, 'I would that they who trouble you would cut the whole thing off' [Gal. 5:12]. And very reasonably, for such a person is venturing on the deeds of murderers, and giving occasion to them that slander God's creation, and opens the mouths of the Manicheans, and is guilty of the same unlawful acts as they that mutilate themselves among the Greeks. For to cut off our members has been from the beginning a work of demoniacal agency, and satanic device, that they may bring up a bad report upon the works of God, that they may mar this living creature, that imputing all not to the choice, but to the nature of our members, the more part of them may sin in security as being irresponsible, and doubly harm this living creature, both by mutilating the members and by impeding the forwardness of the free choice in behalf of good deeds" (ibid., 62:3).

[On sterilization] "Observe how bitterly he [Paul] speaks against their deceivers....'I would that they which trouble you would cut the whole thing off' [Gal. 5:12]....On this account he curses them, and his meaning is as follows: 'For them I have no concern, "A man that is heretical after the first and second admonition refuse" [Titus 3:10]. If they will, let them not only be circumcised but mutilated.' Where then are those who dare to mutilate [sterilize] themselves, seeing that they draw down the apostolic curse, and accuse the workmanship of God, and take part with the Manichees?" (*Commentary on Galatians* 5:12 [AD 395]).

▶ **Jerome** *Late fourth century theologian known for his works on the Bible; d.420.*

"But I wonder why he [the heretic Jovinian] set Judah and Tamar before us for an example, unless perchance even harlots give him pleasure; or Onan, who was slain because he grudged his brother's seed. Does he imagine that we approve of any sexual intercourse except for the procreation of children?" (*Against Jovinian* 1:19 [AD 393]).

"You may see a number of women who are widows before they are wives. Others, indeed, will drink sterility [oral contraceptives] and murder a man not yet born, [and some commit abortion]" (*Letters* 22:13 [AD 396]).

▶ **Augustine** *Well-known and highly prolific theologian, convert, and bishop. His writings include Confessions, The City of God, De Trinitate, and hundreds of other influential works. He also fought against a number of heresies; 354-430.*

"This proves that you [Manicheans] approve of having a wife, not for the procreation of children, but for the gratification of passion. In marriage, as the marriage law declares, the man and woman come together for the procreation of children. Therefore, whoever makes the procreation of children a greater sin than copulation, forbids marriage and makes the woman not a wife but a mistress, who for some gifts presented to her is joined to the man to gratify his passion" (*The Morals of the Manichees* 18:65 [AD 388]).

"You [Manicheans] make your Auditors adulterers of their wives when they take care lest the women with whom they copulate conceive. They take wives according to the laws of matrimony by tablets announcing that the marriage is contracted to procreate children; and then, fearing because of your law [against childbearing]...they copulate in a shameful union only to satisfy lust for their wives. They are unwilling to have children, on whose account alone marriages are made. How is it, then, that you are not those prohibiting marriage, as the Apostle predicted of you so long ago [1 Tim. 4:1-4], when you try to take from marriage what marriage is? When this is taken away, husbands are shameful lovers, wives are harlots, bridal chambers are brothels, fathers-in-law are pimps" (*Against Faustus* 15:7 [AD 400]).

"For thus the eternal law, that is, the will of God creator of all creatures, taking counsel for the conservation of natural order, not to serve lust, but to see to the preservation of the race, permits the delight of mortal flesh to be released from the control of reason in copulation only to propagate progeny" (ibid., 22:30).

"For necessary sexual intercourse for begetting [children] is alone worthy of marriage. But that which goes beyond this necessity no longer follows reason but lust. And yet it pertains to the character of marriage ...to yield it to the partner lest by fornication the other sin damnably [through adultery]....[T]hey [must] not turn away from them the mercy of God...by changing the natural use into that which is against nature, which is more damnable when it is done in the case of husband or wife. For, whereas that natural use, when it pass beyond the compact of marriage, that is, beyond the necessity of begetting [children], is pardonable in the case of a wife, damnable in the case of a harlot; that which is against nature is execrable when done in the case of a harlot, but more execrable in the case of a wife. Of so great power is the ordinance of the Creator, and the order of creation, that . . . when the man shall wish to use a body part of the wife not allowed for this purpose [orally or anally consummated sex], the wife is more shameful, if she suffer it to take place in her own case, than if in the case of another woman" (*The Good of Marriage* 11-12 [AD 401]).

"I am supposing, then, although you are not lying [with your wife] for the sake of procreating offspring, you are not for the sake of lust obstructing their procreation by an evil prayer or an evil deed. Those who do this, although they are called husband and wife, are not; nor do they retain any reality of marriage, but with a respectable name cover a shame. Sometimes this lustful cruelty, or cruel lust, comes to this, that they even procure poisons of sterility [oral contraceptives] . . . Assuredly if both husband and wife are like this, they are not married, and if they were like this from the beginning they come together not joined in matrimony but in seduction. If both are not like this, I dare to say that either the wife is in a fashion the harlot of her husband or he is an adulterer with his own wife" (*Marriage and Concupiscence* 1:15:17 [AD 419]).

▶ Caesarius of Arles *French bishop and theologian; 470-543.*

"Who is he who cannot warn that no woman may take a potion [an oral contraceptive] so that she is unable to conceive or condemns in herself the nature which God willed to be fecund? As often as she could have conceived or given birth, of that many homicides she will be held guilty, and, unless she undergoes suitable penance, she will be damned by eternal death in hell. If a women does not wish to have children, let her enter into a religious agreement with her husband; for chastity is the sole sterility [i.e., postponement of children] of a Christian woman" (*Sermons* 1:12 [AD 522]).

Review Questions

1. What forms did contraception take in the days of the Church Fathers?

2. To what other sins do the Church Fathers compare contraception?

3. What do the Church Fathers say about sterilization?

4. What motives do the Church Fathers identify for the use of contraception by the people of their time? Are these motives different from today's?

Discussion Questions

1. Why is it important to establish the continuity of the Church's teaching on contraception and procreation?

2. Many of the Church Fathers were forceful and vituperative in their condemnation of contraception. What should our tone be when addressing this issue with others? When are we too forceful and when are we not forceful enough?

Chapter 4
Modern Magisterial Teachings

"…any use whatsoever of matrimony exercised in such a way that the act is deliberately frustrated in its natural power to generate life is an offense against the law of God and of nature…"

Pope Pius XI, *Casti Connubii*

(*On Christian Marriage*)

What has the Magisterium said about contraception?

As successors to the Apostles, the Pope and the College of Bishops are commissioned with the office of authoritatively teaching and sanctifying the Church. Often times this office is exercised to give definition to the Church's teaching when its tenets are challenged. Since the time of the Lambeth conference, a 1930 Anglican conference that relaxed what had been a universal condemnation of contraception by Christians, the Church has been called upon numerous times to clarify and reiterate the Church's doctrine on the issue of contraception. In doing so, the Church does not invent new doctrines but rather affirms anew what it has always believed.

▶ Pope Pius XI, Casti Connubii (1930) Encyclical

> "But no reason, however grave, may be put forward by which anything intrinsically against nature may become conformable to nature and morally good. Since, therefore, the conjugal act is destined primarily by nature for the begetting of children, those who in exercising it deliberately frustrate its natural power and purpose sin against nature and commit a deed which is shameful and intrinsically vicious.
>
> Small wonder, therefore, if Holy Writ bears witness that the Divine Majesty regards with greatest detestation this horrible crime and at times has punished it with death. As St. Augustine notes, 'Intercourse even with one's legitimate wife is unlawful and wicked where the conception of the offspring is prevented. Onan, the son of Judah, did this and the Lord killed him for it.'
>
> Since, therefore, openly departing from the uninterrupted Christian tradition some recently have judged it possible solemnly to declare another doctrine regarding this question, the Catholic Church, to whom God has entrusted the defense of the integrity and purity of morals, standing erect in the midst of the moral ruin which surrounds her, in order that she may preserve the chastity of the nuptial union from being defiled by this foul stain, raises her voice in token of her divine ambassadorship and through our mouth proclaims anew: *any use whatsoever of matrimony exercised in such a way that the act is deliberately frustrated in its natural power to generate life is an offense against the law of God and of nature, and those who indulge in such are branded with the guilt of a grave sin.*

We admonish, therefore, priests who hear confessions and others who have the care of souls, in virtue of our supreme authority and in our solicitude for the salvation of souls, not to allow the faithful entrusted to them to err regarding this most grave law of God; much more, that they keep themselves immune from such false opinions, in no way conniving in them. If any confessor or pastor of souls, which may God forbid, lead the faithful entrusted to him into these errors or should at least confirm them by approval or by guilty silence, let him be mindful of the fact that he must render a strict account to God, the Supreme Judge, for the betrayal of his sacred trust, and let him take to himself the words of Christ: 'They are blind and leaders of the blind: and if the blind lead the blind, both fall into the pit'" (54-57).

Did you know…?

"In 1995, the percentage of Catholics using contraception was higher than for the non-Catholic population, 70% vs. 64.2%" (*CCL Family Foundations*, Vol.28, No.2, Sept.-Oct. 2001).

▶ Pope Pius XII Address to Italian Midwives (1951)

"[E]very attempt of either husband or wife in the performance of the conjugal act or in the development of its natural consequences which aims at depriving it of its inherent force and hinders the procreation of new life is immoral; and no 'indication' or need can turn an act which is intrinsically immoral into a moral and lawful one. The precept is in full force today as in the past, and it will be so in the future as well and always, because it is not due to a simple human fancy but is the expression of a natural and divine law."

▶ Pope John XXIII, Mater et Magistra (1961)

"We must solemnly proclaim that human life is transmitted by means of the family, and the family is based upon a marriage which is one and indissoluble and, with respect to Christians, raised to the dignity of a sacrament. The transmission of human life is the result of a personal and conscious act, and, as such, is subject to the all-holy, inviolable and immutable laws of God, which no man may ignore or disobey. He is not therefore permitted to use certain ways and means which are allowable in the propagation of plant and animal life.

Human life is sacred—all men must recognize that fact. From its very inception it reveals the creating hand of God. Those who violate His laws not only offend the divine majesty and degrade themselves and humanity, they also sap the vitality of the political community of which they are members.

A provident God grants sufficient means to the human race to find a dignified solution to the problems attendant upon the transmission of human life. But these problems can become difficult of solution, or even insoluble, if man, led astray in mind and perverted in will, turns to such means as are opposed to right reason, and seeks ends that are contrary to his social nature and the intentions of Providence" (193, 194, 199).

▶ The Second Vatican Council, Gaudium et Spes (1965)

"The sexual characteristics of man and the human faculty of reproduction wonderfully exceed the dispositions of lower forms of life. Hence the acts themselves which are proper to conjugal love and which are exercised in accord with genuine human dignity must be honored with great reverence. Hence when there is question of harmonizing conjugal love with the responsible transmission of life, the moral aspects of any procedure do not depend solely on sincere intentions or on an evaluation of motives, but must be determined by objective standards. These, based on the nature of the human person and his acts, preserve the full sense of mutual self-giving and human procreation in the context of true love. Such a goal cannot be achieved unless the virtue of conjugal chastity is sincerely practiced. Relying on these principles, sons of *the Church may not undertake methods of birth control which are found blameworthy by the teaching authority of the Church in its unfolding of the divine law.*

All should be persuaded that human life and the task of transmitting it are not realities bound up with this world alone. Hence they cannot be measured or perceived only in terms of it, but always have a bearing on the eternal destiny of men" (51).

Bishops Speak

Objective Standards and Freedom of Conscience

Catholics, like all people, are always obligated to follow their consciences—on birth control and every other matter. But that's not where

---

[18] See *Catechism of the Catholic Church* (CCC) number 2370.

the problem lies. The problem lies in the formation of one's conscience. A conscientious person seeks to do good and avoid evil. Seeing the difference between good and evil, though, can sometimes be difficult. As Pope John Paul II has said, the basic moral law is written in the human heart because we're created in the image and likeness of God. But we bear the wounds of original sin, which garbles the message and dims our ability to judge and act according to truth.

Truth is objective. In other words, it's real; independent of us; and exists whether we like it or not. Therefore, conscience can't invent right and wrong. Rather, conscience is called to discover the truth of right and wrong, and then to submit personal judgments to the truth once it is found. Church teaching on the regulation of births, like all her moral teachings, is a sure guide for forming our consciences according to the truth. For we have the certainty of faith, as Vatican II reminds us, that the teachings of the Church on matters of faith and morals are "not the mere word of men, but truly the word of God" (Lumen Gentium 12). Too often, we use "conscience" as a synonym for private preference; a kind of pious alibi for doing what we want or taking the easy road. We only end up hurting others and ourselves.
Charles J. Chaput, O.F.M., Archbishop of Philadelphia, *Of Human Life*

…in their manner of acting, spouses should be aware that they cannot proceed arbitrarily. They must always be governed according to a conscience dutifully conformed to the divine law itself, and should be submissive toward the Church's teaching office, which authentically interprets that law in the light of the Gospel. That divine law reveals and protects the integral meaning of conjugal love and impels it toward a truly human fulfillment.
Vatican II, *Gaudium et Spes* 50

▶ Pope Paul VI, Humanae Vitae (1968)

In conformity with these landmarks in the human and Christian vision of marriage, we must once again declare that the direct interruption of the generative process already begun, and, above all, directly willed and procured abortion, even if for therapeutic reasons, are to be absolutely excluded as licit means of regulating birth.

Equally to be excluded, as the teaching authority of the Church has frequently declared, is direct sterilization, whether perpetual or temporary, whether of the man or of the woman. *Similarly excluded is every action which, either in anticipation of the conjugal* act, or in its accomplishment, or in the development of its natural consequences, proposes, whether as an end or as a means, to render procreation impossible.[18]

To justify conjugal acts made intentionally infecund, one cannot invoke as valid reasons the lesser evil, or the fact that such acts would constitute a whole together with the fecund acts already performed or to follow later, and hence would share in one and the same moral goodness. In truth, if it is sometimes licit to tolerate a lesser evil in order to avoid a greater evil or to promote a greater good, it is not licit, even for the gravest reasons, to do evil so that good may follow therefrom; that is, to make into the object of a positive act of the will something which is intrinsically disorder, and hence unworthy of the human person, even when the intention is to safeguard or promote individual, family or social well-being. Consequently it is an error to think that a conjugal act which is deliberately made infecund and so is intrinsically dishonest could be made honest and right by the ensemble of a fecund conjugal life (14).

Sterilization: Perpetual Contraception...

"Equally to be excluded, as the teaching authority of the Church has frequently declared, is direct sterilization, whether permanent or temporary, whether of the man or of the woman" (*Humanae Vitae* 14).

"When they have two or more children, 55% of Catholic parents are sterilized" (*CCL Family Foundations* Vol. 28, No. 2, Sept.-Oct. 2001).

▶ Pope John Paul II, Familiaris Consortio (1981)

When couples, by means of recourse to contraception, separate these two meanings [unitive and procreative] that God the creator has inscribed in the being of man and woman and in the dynamism of their sexual communion, they act as "arbiters" of the divine plan and they "manipulate" and degrade human sexuality and with it themselves and their married partner by altering its value of "total" self-giving. Thus the innate language that expresses the total reciprocal self-giving of husband and wife is overlaid, through contraception, by an objectively contradictory language, namely, that of not giving oneself totally to the other. This leads not only to a positive refusal to be open to life, but also to a falsification of the inner truth of conjugal love, which is called upon to give itself in personal totality (32).

In Vitro Fertilization & Artificial Reproductive Technologies

Techniques that entail the *dissociation of husband and wife, by the intrusion of a person other than the couple* (donation of sperm or ovum, surrogate uterus) are gravely immoral. These techniques (heterologous artificial insemination and fertilization) infringe the child's right to be born of a father and mother known to him and bound to each other by marriage. They betray the spouses' "right to become a father and a mother only through each other" (CCC 2376).

Techniques involving only the married couple (homologous artificial insemination and fertilization) are perhaps less reprehensible, yet remain morally unacceptable. They dissociate the sexual act from the procreative act. The act which brings the child into existence is no longer an act by which two persons give themselves to one another, but one that "entrusts the life and identity of the embryo into the power of doctors and biologists and establishes the domination of technology over the origin and destiny of the human person. Such a relationship of domination is in itself contrary to the dignity and equality that must be common to parents and children" [*Donum Vitae* II,5]. "Under the moral aspect procreation is deprived of its proper perfection when it is not willed as the fruit of the *conjugal act*, that is to say, of the specific act of the spouses' union…Only respect for the link between the meanings of the conjugal act and respect for the unity of the human being make possible procreation in conformity with the dignity of the person"[*Donum Vitae* II,4] (CCC 2377).

Review Questions

1. Which magisterial statement teaches that contraception is a "grave sin"?

2. To whom is Pope Pius XI referring in *Casti Connubii* when he quotes the words of Christ: "They are blind and leaders of the blind; and if the blind lead the blind, both fall into the pit"?

3. Pius XII's Address to Italian Midwives teaches that the Church's teaching on contraception and procreation is an expression of what?

4. Pope John XXIII teaches in *Mater et Magistra* that human life is transmitted by what means? What means in his teaching is not permitted?

5. Gaudium et Spes teaches that the moral aspects of procreation do not depend solely on what?

6. What does Charles J. Chaput, Archbishop of Denver, say is too often used as a synonym for private preference?

7. What explanation does Pope Paul VI give in *Humanae Vitae* for his assertion that one cannot invoke "the lesser evil" as a valid reason for using contraception?

8. Why is in vitro fertilization and artificial insemination morally impermissible? (Consider both homologous methods—methods performed between spouses—and heterologous methods—procedures that entail the involvement of a person from outside the couple).

9. According to *Familiaris Consortio,* why is the use of contraception an "objectively contradictory language"?

Discussion Question

Why do you think so many Catholics choose sterilization (vasectomy or tubal ligation) as a means of contraception? What should Catholics who have been sterilized do to repent of, or make reparation for, this wrongdoing?

Chapter 5
Natural Family Planning

"In its true meaning, responsible procreation requires couples to be obedient to the Lord's call and to act as faithful interpreters of his plan. This happens when the family is generously open to new lives, and when couples maintain an attitude of openness and service to life, even if, for serious reasons and in respect for the moral law, they choose to avoid a new birth for the time being or indefinitely. The moral law obliges them in every case to control the impulse of instinct and passion, and to respect the biological laws inscribed in their person. It is precisely this respect which makes legitimate, at the service of responsible procreation, the *use of natural methods of regulating fertility.*"

Pope John Paul II, *The Gospel of Life* **97**

What is Natural Family Planning?

Natural Family Planning (NFP) is a comprehensive acceptance of the divine gift of fertility within marriage, wherein the couple monitors their fertility to determine fertile and non-fertile phases for the purpose of either achieving or postponing pregnancy. It is not to be confused with the older and significantly less effective "calendar rhythm method" which estimates and projects the couple's fertile and non-fertile phases by observing when these phases occurred in previous cycles.

The greater effectiveness of NFP is due to a much more precise and systematic approach in which, *depending on the method*, couples observe changes in the woman's cervical mucus, temperature changes and/or other signs to determine fertile and non-fertile phases. Since both cervical mucus and temperature are responsive to the chemical/hormonal changes that regulate fertility, NFP users are able to accurately determine when they are fertile and when they are not. The outmoded calendar rhythm method was more of an educated guess that relied heavily on the often erroneous assumption that fertility cycles are the same from month to month.

NFP users are able to determine their fertility by simply observing their cervical mucus and/or temperature and charting it. The process takes only minutes a day, and with the observance of a few simple rules yields an effectiveness rate for postponing pregnancy equal to or better than any artificial contraceptive methods. In fact the Couple to Couple League, an international Natural Family Planning organization in Cincinnati, Ohio, cites numerous studies, including one conducted by the U.S. government, that show the Sympto-Thermal Method of NFP, which combines temperature and mucus observations, can be used at the 99% level of effectiveness for postponing pregnancy. It is also highly effective for *achieving* pregnancy and is used by many couples as a means of overcoming difficulties conceiving.

What are the advantages of Natural Family Planning?

❶ **Natural Family Planning is safe, healthy, and inexpensive.**

Natural Family Planning does nothing to chemically alter a woman's natural cycle and it makes use of no invasive or prophylactic measures such as IUDs, diaphragms, condoms, and spermicides to interfere with a woman's fertility. There is no cost to NFP except a meager fee for classes, a basal thermometer, and charts. Mucus-only NFP users pay only for charts. Compare this to the cost of pills, condoms, diaphragms, injections, doctor visits, treatment for side effects, chemicals, and implants, and the cost difference is obvious.

❷ **NFP is effective for avoiding AND achieving pregnancy.**

NFP meets or exceeds the effectiveness rates of all contraceptive methods if used properly. In fact, all the methods of NFP can be used at the 99% level of effectiveness to postpone or avoid pregnancy.[19] "Several well-designed trials by the World Health Organization have shown that Natural Family Planning…has had an effectiveness rate when used correctly that is better than OCPs (oral contraceptive pills), that is, less than a 3% rate of pregnancies per year… One of the largest trials (of 19,843 women performed by the World Health Organization in India) showed the failure rate to be 0.2 pregnancies per 100 women yearly—a rate that is significantly better than almost all artificial methods of contraception."[20] Some simple rules must be followed to achieve this level of effectiveness but this is true of artificial contraception as well. The misuse rates of condoms and pills are startlingly high and typically exceed those of NFP users.[21] One distinct advantage of NFP over contraception is that it is immediately reversible unlike IUDs, injections, implants, and sterilization.

❸ **NFP contributes to the health and welfare of the marriage.**

Unlike contraception, which acts as an inhibitor of one's natural fertility, NFP keeps it intact and works within it. In this way it is not a rejection of the gifts that husband and wife have to offer each other. The marital embrace is a complete gift of self to one's spouse—nothing is held back. Yet these gifts are not reducible to a sharing in the physiological aspects of fertility. The marital act is a visible sign of the reality that two have become one; that in the covenant of marriage each spouse belongs fully to the other—*nothing is held back*. In the act of making love, spouses say with their bodies what they intend with their hearts. If fertility is withheld, this covenant expression is weakened if not wholly disintegrated. It becomes a conspicuous reservation in which, in keeping with the expression "actions speak louder than

---

[19] Kippley, John & Sheila. *The Art of Natural Family Planning*. The Couple to Couple League Intl (CCL). Cincinnati: 1996; p. 3.
[20] Kahlenborn, Chris, M.D., *Breast Cancer: Its Link to Abortion and the Birth Control Pill*, One More Soul, Dayton, Ohio, 2000, p.39.
[21] Kippley, p. 146. The Guttmacher Institute, a research institute affiliated with Planned Parenthood, cites failure rates for the condom as high as 18.5% (low 9.8%), and for the Pill failure rates as high as 8.7% (low 3.8%).

words," spouses say, "you can have all of me except my power to give life." It is not hard to understand why many married people feel used, even betrayed, by contraceptive sex; for implicit in this mutual withholding of self is a mutual *rejection*. Sex that does not accept the fullness of the other can easily become self-directed, reducing sex to a matter of self-indulgence and physical gratification, so much so that it becomes a wedge instead of a bond. Perhaps this is why divorce rates for NFP users are between 1/10 and 1/25 of the overall divorce rate in the United States in the 90s.[22] Indeed, a study conducted by the *Family of Americas Foundation* **found only 18 divorces among 505 couples, a rate of 3.6%!**[23]

❹ NFP is consistent with the life of faith.

There is no greater happiness and fulfillment than a life lived in and through God. Eliminating obstacles to this relationship is a positive choice, freeing us to love as fully as possible. The Church teaches against contraception not to impose arbitrary prohibitions, but to safeguard marriage and to deepen the expression of marital love.

Bishops Speak

Responding to the objection that contraception and Natural Family Planning are essentially the same...

Most Reverend Charles J. Chaput, O.F.M., Cap., Archbishop of Philadelphia

Objection: I still don't see the big difference between a couple using "artificial" birth control and a couple using "natural" family planning. Don't both couples have the same intention, and isn't this what determines morality?

Response: It's hard to see the difference when the emphasis is placed on "artificial" versus "natural" methods. People rightly point out that many things we use are artificial but not immoral. So it's important to realize that the Church doesn't oppose artificial birth control *be-*

---

[22] Kippley, p. 288. The Couple to Couple League (CCL) estimates the divorce rate among NFP users at between 2% and 5% as opposed to the general divorce rate of approximately 50% in the U.S. in the early 90s.

[23] Wilson, Mercedes. "The Practice of Natural Family Planning Versus the Use of Artificial Birth Control: Family, Sexual and Moral Issues" *Catholic Social Scientist Review,* Vol. VI. 2002

cause it's artificial. Rather, what the Church opposes is *any* method of birth control which is *contraceptive*, whether artificial devices, pills, etc. are used or not.

Contraception is the choice, by any means, to *sterilize a given act of intercourse*. In other words, a contracepting couple chooses to engage in intercourse and, knowing that it may result in a new life, they intentionally and willfully suppress their fertility. Herein lies a key distinction: Natural Family Planning (NFP) *is in no way contraceptive*. The choice to *abstain* from a fertile act of intercourse is completely different from the willful choice to *sterilize* a fertile act of intercourse. NFP simply accepts from God's hand the natural cycle of infertility that He has built into the nature of woman.

Regarding the issue of intention: Yes, both couples may have the same *end* in mind—to avoid pregnancy. But the *means* to achieve their common goal are not alike. Take, for example, two students, each of whom intends to excel in school. Obviously that's a very good intention. With the same goal in mind, one studies diligently. The other cheats on every test. The point is, the end doesn't justify the means—in getting an education, in regulating births, or in anything else.

Of Human Life: A Pastoral Letter to the People of God of Northern Colorado on the Truth and Meaning of Married Love: July 22, 1998.

Most Reverend John J. Myers, Archbishop of Newark

In contraceptive intercourse the married couple is saying, "We know that our love for each other can create a new life. We do not want this new life at this time. Therefore we will, by a directly willed positive act, destroy that creative part of our love. Though our bodies are saying we love each other completely, we do not love our fertility at this time. Thus we will sterilize our love."

Trust the Truth: A Symposium on the Twentieth Anniversary of the Encyclical Humanae Vitae. The Pope John Center, Braintree, Massachusetts: 1991; p.73.

Natural Family Planning: A Secret No More!
Most Reverend John C. Favalora, Former Archbishop of Miami

Some people call it the best kept secret in the Catholic Church. Here in the Archdiocese of Miami, we're determined to change that. I am referring to Natural Family Planning, an effective, totally natural, side-effect-free method of postponing or planning a pregnancy, one that is scientifically proven and in keeping with the moral teachings of the Church.

Natural Family Planning is not the old, unreliable "rhythm" method which hinged on the calendar to predict when a woman was fertile. Through Natural Family Planning, a woman tracks her fertility by observing the physical changes in her body: chiefly the characteristics of the mucus discharged from the cervix and her body temperature when she awakens in the morning.

Natural Family Planning actually is the generic term for several natural methods of fertility awareness, two of which are taught in the archdiocese. One is known as the Ovulation Method because it requires couples to chart only the characteristics of the cervical mucus, the chief indicator of ovulation. The other is called the Sympto-Thermal Method because it incorporates other signs of ovulation, including the woman's basal body temperature and the condition of her cervix.

Both methods have a scientific basis. They were developed by medical professionals and have been tested in health trials worldwide. They can be used by women with both regular and irregular menstrual cycles. And they are just as effective for women who are breast-feeding or undergoing menopause, since they track the hormonal changes that naturally occur in a woman's body. How effective are they? Medical professionals have relied on them for years to pinpoint the moment of ovulation in women who have difficulty getting pregnant.

Amazingly, these methods of Natural Family Planning were developed in the 1960s—around the same time as the Pill, which garnered bigger headlines. The outcry against rhythm also caused a majority of Catholics to reject any "natural" method, although thousands are re-discovering them today.

True, these methods require couples to abstain from sexual intercourse during certain times of a woman's cycle, if they wish to avoid pregnancy. Self-discipline is not popular in our "instant" age. But we all must set limits and abstain from certain activities at certain times in our lives. Alcohol, chocolate, food, sleep or even exercise may bring us pleasure, but we cannot indulge non-stop in any of them. Why should sex be different?

Couples who use natural methods of family planning report greater satisfaction and increased pleasure during those times when they can engage in sexual activity, referring to them as mini-honeymoons. They also report better communication between the spouses and an increased sense of intimacy, since we all know that men tend to equate sex with intimacy while women define it in broader terms.

The fact that Natural Family Planning methods require the cooperation of both husband and wife is even a selling point for feminists, who lament that the advent of the Pill has placed the burden of birth control squarely on the shoulders of women. Best of all, women who use natural methods don't have to deal with the negative side effects and possible long-term health consequences of the Pill or other barrier methods.

So why don't more couples use Natural Family Planning? Because they don't know about it. The Church itself has failed to teach about the effectiveness and moral acceptability of these methods.

That is why, when I promulgated new marriage guidelines two years ago, I instructed that a section on Natural Family Planning be added to all the marriage preparation courses required by the archdiocese. I want all the Catholic couples getting married in South Florida to know about these methods and be encouraged to use them, since they are not only healthier than the artificial ones, they are also morally correct.
[*Reprinted with permission, CatholicExchange.com*]

Family Planning: An International Perspective
Dr. John C. Wilke, MD

Friends, if there's one country in the world that has been simply overwhelmed with foreign aid workers seeking to reduce its population, it's Bangladesh. This nation is one of the poorest in the world and one of the more densely populated. As a result of this, major international agencies have flooded the country with workers, bringing with them various contraceptives. These workers are paid per capita, that is, depending upon how many families they get to use contraceptives.

Understand, now, there is almost no religious objection to using contraceptives in Bangladesh, as the overwhelming majority of its population is Muslim and Hindu. In light of this, I was rather surprised to learn that many women in Bangladesh, when offered the options, select Natural Family Planning over artificial means of contraception.

As most of you know, international family planning and population control agencies have held that the only realistic option for poor, uneducated women in the developing world is artificial contraception, and they much prefer the long-term methods of intrauterine devices and chemical and surgical castration.

But Dr. Hanna Klaus, in a recent article in the British medical journal *The Lancet* (January 26, 2002) brings us a different story. It is of the widespread popularity and effectiveness of Natural Family Planning. She says that the international agencies disregard the actual capabilities, intelligence, and motivation of poor women. They illustrate an elitist's condescension and treat women more as veterinary medicine would.

Dr. Klaus offered Natural Family Planning through *Caritas*, a Catholic agency, but only one-third of the women using it were Catholic; the rest were Muslim and Hindu. She gives considerable detail showing that the effectiveness of this method is superior, in most cases, to the record of artificial means of planning the family.

She described instances in which paid family planning officials followed the Natural Family Planning teachers on their rounds, because the paid officials had quotas to fill in order to keep their jobs. They would record the women who accepted the Natural Family Planning and then would later return to try to convince them to switch back to artificial means.

Dr. Klaus, in her article, states that the Bangladesh experience shows that NFP should be considered a modern method of family planning, because it works and works very effectively. For the developing world, she believes it should be considered the first and most appropriate method of family planning.

The reasons she gives are—it costs nothing; it results in no serious medical complications but, most importantly, it shows respect for people. Her conclusion—when people are respected, they respond.
Natural Family Planning in Bangladesh, Life Issues No.33-6. Reprinted with permission www.lifeissues.org.

Review Questions

1. Natural Family Planning should not be confused with what other less effective natural method?

2. How effective is Natural Family Planning for postponing pregnancy?

3. What is the divorce rate of NFP users compared to that of the general population?

Discussion Questions

1. Why do you think the divorce rate is lower for NFP users than for the general population?

2. A. For NFP users: Share your experience with NFP.

    B. For Married/Engaged couples hesitant to use NFP: What are your doubts and concerns about using Natural Family Planning?

    C. For unmarried/non-engaged singles: Do you know couples that use NFP? If so, what is your impression of its effects on their marriages? If you know married couples that don't use NFP, why do you think they don't use it?

Chapter 6
The Connection between Contraception and Abortion

"It may be that many people use contraception with a view to excluding the subsequent temptation of abortion. But the negative values inherent in the 'contraceptive mentality'—which is very different from responsible parenthood, lived in respect for the full truth of the conjugal act—are such that they in fact strengthen this temptation when an unwanted life is conceived."

Pope John Paul II, *The Gospel of Life* **13**

What is the connection between contraception and abortion?

In a culture that so often justifies the means of an act by its end, it is not surprising that contraception and abortion would have a close association. For behind both contraception and abortion is the contention that in order to avoid pregnancy artificial and intrusive means may be used to thwart the body's natural reproductive capacity. While abortion and contraception are separate evils, they are both the product of man's desire to countermand God's control over human sexuality and its natural consequences. Let us consider three illustrations of this relationship.

❶ Contraceptives can be abortifacients.

"Every form of chemical birth control has the power to cause early abortions. This applies to every form of the Pill, to implants such as Norplant and to injections such as Depo-Provera."[24] In the not uncommon case of breakthrough ovulation, many such contraceptives have a mode of action that makes the uterine lining inhospitable to the newly conceived child, potentially causing abortion. Modern research has shown "a 'breakthrough ovulation' rate of 4.7%" for the Pill.[25] Studies of Norplant have shown breakthrough ovulation increased with each year of use: "…it was noted that the breakthrough ovulation rate in the first year of use was 11%, but increased dramatically after that year, so that a 7-year average yielded an annual breakthrough ovulation rate of 44%."[26] Even if only a fraction of these "breakthrough ovulations" resulted in conception, the result would be thousands of abortions, given the millions of women who use birth control.

❷ Abortion has become a form of birth control.

The Supreme Court decision, *Planned Parenthood v. Casey*, points out this disturbing phenomenon:

> [I]n some critical respects the abortion decision is of the same character as the decision to use contraception…for two decades of economic and social developments, people have organized intimate relationships and made choices that define their views of themselves and their places in society, in reliance on the availability of abortion in the event that contraception should fail.[27]

---

[24] Kippley, John & Sheila. *The Art of Natural Family Planning*, Fourth Edition. The Couple to Couple League. Cincinnati, Ohio: 1996, p.9.
[25] Ibid., p.9.
[26] Kahlenborn, Chris, M.D., *Breast Cancer: Its Link to Abortion and the Birth Control Pill*, One More Soul, Dayton, Ohio, 2000, p.324-325.
[27] Smith, Janet. "The Connection between Contraception and Abortion." One More Soul. Dayton, Ohio.

Repeat abortions provide further evidence that abortion has become a form of backup contraception:
- In 1994-95, nearly half (45 percent) of women obtaining abortions in the U.S. had previously aborted one or more times.
- The proportion of women who have had previous abortions reaches 60 percent among women 30 and older.
- By 1987, 15.1 million women had *at least* one abortion since states began to legalize abortion in 1967. That figure was projected to be 17.8 million by the end of 1990.[28]

❸ Abortion flows from an anti-conception mentality.

Pope John Paul II explains this connection in his landmark encyclical *The Gospel of Life*:

It is frequently asserted that *contraception*, if made safe and available to all, is the most effective remedy against abortion. The Catholic Church is then accused of actually promoting abortion, because she obstinately continues to teach the moral unlawfulness of contraception. When looked at carefully, this objection is clearly unfounded. It may be that many people use contraception with a view to excluding the subsequent temptation of abortion. But the negative values inherent in the "contraceptive mentality"—which is very different from responsible parenthood, lived in respect for the full truth of the conjugal act—are such that they in fact strengthen this temptation when an unwanted life is conceived. Indeed, the pro-abortion culture is especially strong precisely where the Church's teaching on contraception is rejected. Certainly, from the moral point of view contraception and abortion are specifically different evils: the former contradicts the full truth of the sexual act as the proper expression of conjugal love, while the latter destroys the life of a human being; the former is opposed to the virtue of chastity in marriage, the latter is opposed to the virtue of justice and directly violates the divine commandment "You shall not kill."

But despite their differences of nature and moral gravity, contraception and abortion are often closely connected, as fruits of the same tree. It is true that in many cases contraception and even abortion are practiced under the pressure of real-life difficulties, which nonetheless can never exonerate from striving to observe God's law fully. Still, in very many other instances such practices are rooted in a hedonistic mentality unwilling to

---

[28] *Family Planning Perspectives* (Alan Guttmacher Institute) 23:75, March/April 1991; 28:140, July/August 1996.

[29] Pope John Paul II. *The Gospel of Life*. Times Books/Random House. New York: 1995, pp. 23-24.

accept responsibility in matters of sexuality, and they imply a self-centered concept of freedom, which regards procreation as an obstacle to personal fulfillment. *The life which could result from a sexual encounter thus becomes an enemy to be avoided at all costs and abortion becomes the only possible decisive response to failed contraception.*

The close connection which exists, in mentality, between the practice of contraception and that of abortion is becoming increasingly obvious. It is being demonstrated in an alarming way by the development of chemical products, intrauterine devices, and vaccines which, distributed with the same ease as contraceptives, really act as abortifacients in the very early stages of the development of the life of the new human being.[29]

Professor Charles Rice puts the abortion–contraception connection this way:

If man (of both sexes) makes himself, through contraception, the arbiter of when life begins, he will predictably make himself the arbiter of when it shall end. Contraception prevents life while abortion kills existing life. But both involve the deliberate separation of the unitive and procreative aspects of sex. A contraceptive society requires abortion as a backup for contraception. The availability of abortion is also a factor in the decision of some to engage in sexual relations without using contraception. And many so-called contraceptives are abortifacient in that they cause the destruction of the developing human being.[30]

Bishops Speak
USCCB

The Church's teaching and pastoral efforts on responsible parenthood are appropriately treated more fully in other documents. However, we address the issue here because some promote wide-spread use of contraception as a means to reduce abortions and even criticize the Church for not accepting this approach.

It is noteworthy that as acceptance and use of contraception have increased in our society, so have acceptance and use of abortion. Couples who unintentionally conceive a child while using contraception are far more likely to resort to abortion than others. Tragically, our society has fallen into a mentality that views children as a burden and invites many to consider abortion as a "backup" to contraceptive failure. This is most obvious in efforts to promote as "emergency contraception" drugs that really act as early abortifacients.

---

[30] Rice, Charles. *The Winning Side: Questions on Living the Culture of Life.* St. Brendan's Institute, Mishawaka, Indiana: 1999, p.112.

> With Pope John Paul II we affirm that contraception and abortion are "specifically different evils," because only "the latter destroys the life of a human being," but that they are also related (*The Gospel of Life*, no. 13). It is important to remember that means that are referred to as "contraceptive" are, in reality, sometimes also abortifacient. An end to abortion will not come from contraceptive campaigns but from a deeper understanding of our human sexuality, and of human life, as sacred gifts deserving our careful stewardship.
>
> *U.S. Conference of Catholic Bishops, Pastoral Plan for Pro-Life Activities, "A Campaign in Support of Life"*

Review Questions

1. How is hormonal birth control abortifacient?

2. What point does Planned Parenthood v. Casey make about the relationship between abortion and contraception?

3. What is Pope John Paul II's explanation for why abortion and contraception are "closely connected, as fruits of the same tree"?

4. The USCCB argues that abortion as a "backup" to failed contraception is most obvious in efforts to promote what?

Discussion Question

A survey released in 1996 by the Alan Guttmacher Institute (the research arm of Planned Parenthood) shows that between 1994-1995, 57.5% of 10,000 abortion patients were using contraception during the month in which they became pregnant. Malcom Potts, the former medical director of the International Planned Parenthood Federation predicted in the same year abortion was legalized, "As people turn to contraception, there well be a rise, not a fall, in the abortion rate." In light of the evidence of the connection between contraception and abortion, why do you think the pro-life movement around the world fails to more widely denounce the use of contraception?

Chapter 7
Authority and Dissent

"Unless a man is able to say to himself, as in the Presence of God, that he must not, and dare not, act upon the Papal injunction, he is bound to obey it and would commit a great sin in disobeying it. Prima facie it is his bounden duty, even from a sentiment of loyalty, to believe the Pope right and to act accordingly..."

Cardinal Newman, *A Letter to the Duke of Norfolk*

Is it okay to dissent from the Church's teaching on contraception?

In a recent RCIA meeting, the topic of contraception arose as part of a discussion of the sixth commandment and chastity. One of the sponsors in our group objected that she considered some of the teachings of the Church optional; that contraception is one of the issues on which she must "agree to disagree" with the Church. Unfortunately this is not uncommon in the Church today, and dissent over the moral teachings of the Church is not limited to contraception. The fact is that the Church's teaching on contraception is authoritative and obligatory, and is supported by the witness of Scripture, Tradition, and the Magisterium. Our acceptance of the Church's teaching inherently transcends obligation, or mere legal observance because (1) the Church is divinely commissioned to shepherd the faithful, and (2) God has exalted marriage as a sacrament that, when lived out according to its proper ends, sanctifies spouses and the whole family of God. We are to embrace our fertility and the gift of children within marriage as key components of complete self-giving love for God and neighbor. Our faithfulness to God's design for human sexuality, in other words, helps us to live our vocation to its fullest, opening for us a more secure pathway to God.

❶ Married couples may not, in the name of autonomy or freedom of conscience, ignore the teaching of the Church on this issue.

> ▶ Vatican II, Pastoral Constitution on the Church in the Modern World 50
>
>> Married people should realize that in their behavior they may not simply follow their own fancy but must be ruled by conscience—and conscience ought to be conformed to the law of God in the light of the teaching authority of the Church, which is the authentic interpreter of divine law. For the divine law throws light on the meaning of married love, protects it and leads it to truly human fulfillment.
>
> ▶ Pope Paul VI, Humanae Vitae 10
>
>> In the task of transmitting life, they are not free, therefore, to proceed at will, as if they could determine with complete autonomy the right paths to follow; but they must conform their actions to the creative intention of God, expressed in the very nature of

marriage and of its acts, and manifested by the constant teaching of the Church.

❷ Married couples cannot practice contraception on the grounds that it is not a grave matter.

▶ Pope Pius XI, Casti Connubii 56

Any use whatsoever of matrimony exercised in such a way that the [sexual] act is deliberately frustrated in its natural power to generate life is an offense against the law of God and of nature, and those who indulge in such are branded with the guilt of grave sin.

▶ Catechism of the Catholic Church 2370-2371

Quoting *Humanae Vitae*, the Catechism teaches, "'every action which, whether in anticipation of the conjugal act, or in its accomplishment, or in the development of its natural consequences, proposes, whether as an end or as a means, to render procreation impossible' is *intrinsically evil*."

Next the Catechism situates the transmission of human life in the context of man's eternal destiny: "Let all be convinced that human life and the duty of transmitting it are not limited by the horizons of this life only; their true evaluation and full significance can be understood only in reference to *man's eternal destiny*."

▶ Pope Paul VI, Humanae Vitae 17

The gravity of an action may be seen, in part, by its consequences:

Upright men can even better convince themselves of the solid grounds on which the teaching of the Church in this field is based, if they care to reflect upon the consequences of methods of artificial birth control. Let them consider, first of all, how wide and easy a road would thus be opened up towards conjugal infidelity and the general lowering of morality. Not much experience is needed in order to know human weakness, and to understand that men—especially the young, who are so vulnerable on this point—have need of encouragement to be faithful to the moral law, so that they must not be offered some easy means of eluding its observance. It is also to be feared that the man, growing used to the employment of anti-conceptive practices, may finally lose respect for the woman and, no longer caring for her physical and psychological equilibrium, may come to the point of considering her as a mere instrument of selfish enjoyment, and no longer as his respected and beloved companion.

Let it be considered also that a dangerous weapon would thus be placed in the hands of those public authorities who take no heed of moral exigencies. Who could blame a government for applying to the solution of the problems of the community those means acknowledged to be licit for married couples in the solution of a family problem? Who will stop rulers from favoring, from even imposing upon their peoples, if they were to consider it necessary, the method of contraception which they judge to be most efficacious? In such a way men, wishing to avoid individual, family, or social difficulties encountered in the observance of the divine law, would reach the point of placing at the mercy of the intervention of public authorities the most personal and most reserved sector of conjugal intimacy.

Consequently, if the mission of generating life is not to be exposed to the arbitrary will of men, one must necessarily recognize insurmountable limits to the possibility of man's domination over his own body and its functions; limits which no man, whether a private individual or one invested with authority, may licitly surpass.

Practicing what we preach...

The transmission of human life is a gift that God takes seriously. For this reason, the Church has taught authoritatively that God's plan for procreation cannot be usurped. To do so would constitute *an act of rebellion*, a form of self-gratification in opposition to God's sovereign will and the authoritative teaching of His holy instrument of salvation, the Church. Dr. John Hardon, author of *The Catholic Catechism* and *Modern Catholic Dictionary* – two of his eighteen books – distills the Church's teaching on the gravity of contraception: "…the deliberate practice of contraception between husband and wife is objectively a mortal sin. Those who persist in its practice are acting contrary to the explicit teaching of the Roman Catholic Church. They may protest that they are Catholic. They may profess to be Catholics. But their conduct belies their profession."[31]

---

[31] *Contraception: Fatal to the Faith*, Trinity Communications, The Catholic Resource Network (CRNET), Manassas, Virginia: 1994.

❸ Counsel from a priest or theologian that contraception is permissible is erroneous.

▶ Pope Pius XI, Casti Connubii 57

> We admonish, therefore, priests who hear confessions and others who have the care of souls, in virtue of our supreme authority and in our solicitude for the salvation of souls, not to allow the faithful entrusted to them to err regarding this most grave law of God; much more, that they keep themselves immune from such false opinions, in no way conniving in them. If any confessor or pastor of souls, which may God forbid, leads the faithful entrusted to him into these errors or should at least confirm them by approval or by guilty silence, let him be mindful of the fact that he must render a strict account to God, the Supreme Judge, for the betrayal of his sacred trust, and let him take to himself the words of Christ: "They are blind and leaders of the blind; and if the blind lead the blind, both fall into the pit."

▶ Pope John Paul II, Conference on Problems of Responsible Procreation, June 5, 1987

> Those who place themselves in open conflict with the law of God, authentically taught by the Church, lead spouses along a false path. What the Church teaches concerning contraception does not pertain to the category of matter open to discussion among theologians. To teach the contrary is to lead the moral conscience of spouses into error.

❹ Spouses may not disobey the Church's teaching on contraception on the grounds that it is not an ex cathedra teaching or that the Church has no authority over this issue.

▶ Vatican II, Dogmatic Constitution on the Church 25

> For the bishops are heralds of the faith, who draw new disciples to Christ; they are authentic teachers, that is, *teachers endowed with the authority of Christ*, who preach to the people assigned to them the faith which is to be believed and applied in practice; and under the light of the holy Spirit they cause that faith to radiate, drawing from the storehouse of revelation new things and old;

they make it bear fruit and they vigilantly ward off whatever errors threaten their flock. Bishops who teach in communion with the Roman Pontiff *are to be respected by all as witnesses of divine and catholic truth*; the faithful, for their part, should concur with their bishop's judgment, made in the name of Christ, in matters of faith and morals, and adhere to it with a religious docility of spirit. This religious docility of the will and intellect must be extended, in a special way, to the authentic teaching authority of the Roman Pontiff, *even when he does not speak ex cathedra*, in such wise, indeed, that his supreme teaching authority be acknowledged with respect....[32]

▶ Pope Paul VI, Humanae Vitae 4

...Jesus Christ when communicating to Peter and to the apostles His divine authority and sending them to teach all nations His commandments, constituted them as guardians and authentic interpreters of all the moral law, not only, that is, of the law of the Gospel, but also of the natural law, which is also an expression of the will of God, the faithful fulfillment of which is equally necessary for salvation.

Conformably to this mission of hers, the Church has always provided–and even more amply in recent times–a coherent teaching concerning both the nature of marriage and the correct use of conjugal rights and the duties of husband and wife...

Review Questions

1. The Pastoral Constitution on the Church in the Modern World (50) teaches that conscience ought to be conformed to what?

2. Pope Paul VI teaches in *Humanae Vitae* that couples must conform their actions to what?

---

[32] Some argue that the teaching of the Catholic Church on contraception is an infallible and irreversible exercise of the Ordinary Magisterium, that is, the general and ordinary teaching authority of the bishops in union with the Pope, due to the universality and endurance of the doctrine as well as the unequivocal quality of its expression. As a component of the Natural Law, the Church's teaching on contraception, defined as infallible or not, is true and binding as are many of the moral laws by which we abide without benefit of solemn definition.

3. The Catechism of the Catholic Church (2371) teaches that the duty of transmitting human life can be understood only in reference to what?

4. In the teaching of Pope Paul VI, what are the four consequences of contraception use?

5. Pope John Paul II taught, at the Conference on Problems of Responsible Procreation, that what the Church teaches concerning contraception does not pertain to what category?

6. The Dogmatic Constitution on the Church, n.25, teaches that the teaching of the Holy Father is to be accepted as authoritative and morally binding even when he does not speak in what way?

Discussion Question

George Weigel, in his book *The Courage to be Catholic* makes the following argument:

> The public controversy over Pope Paul VI's encyclical *Humanae Vitae*, was perhaps the crucial moment in the formation of a culture of dissent that would influence the Catholic Church in the United States for the rest of the twentieth century.

Why is our assent to or rejection of the Church's teaching on contraception crucial to our general acceptance of the Catholic faith?

Chapter 8
The Blessings of Children

Thus amongst the blessings of marriage, the child holds the first place. And indeed the Creator of the human race Himself, Who in His goodness wishes to use men as His helpers in the propagation of life, taught this when, instituting marriage in Paradise, He said to our first parents, and through them to all future spouses: "Increase and multiply, and fill the earth." As St. Augustine admirably deduces from the words of the holy Apostle Saint Paul to Timothy when he says: "The Apostle himself is therefore a witness that marriage is for the sake of generation: 'I wish,' he says, 'young girls to marry.' And, as if someone said to him, 'Why?,' he immediately adds: 'To bear children, to be mothers of families'…[I]t is easily seen *how great a gift of divine goodness and how remarkable a fruit of marriage are children born by the omnipotent power of God through the cooperation of those bound in wedlock."*

Pope Pius XI, Casti Connubii 11&12

How are children a blessing?

The Church's teaching on contraception is not just a prohibition but a calling to the joy of parenthood. Procreation of children, far greater than an obligation, is an outpouring of God's love to spouses, who in turn pour out their love to their children. Parents accordingly become mediators, instruments, and ministers of God's love. This sharing in God's love of His children, as is true of all instances in which we share in the administration of God's gifts, heightens our dignity, conforms us to Christ, and deepens our self-knowledge.

The transmission of human life, a prerogative so cherished by God that it has been entrusted only to the covenantal union of man and wife, is essential to the *vocation* of marriage.[32] Yes, marriage is a vocation raised by Christ to the level of a sacrament. Like all the sacraments, marriage is an encounter with Christ that nourishes one's own earthly pilgrimage as God's life and love (grace) is poured into one's soul. Yet God in his abundance fills the soul to overflowing, surging beyond our boundaries so that we become vessels of his love. In so doing, we become living images of Christ in the world.

Children are the incarnation of married love; the material overflowing of two becoming one. Love is *always* life-giving, *always* open to the other, *always* expansive. Those who love find no greater joy than to extend love to others. Children are the natural extension of the love of spouses—the visible sign of the fruitfulness of self-emptying love—and a means of ever deepening joy in marriage.

This is not to say that having children will create a perpetual state of marital bliss. Children involve sacrifice, *but* sacrifice is the fuel of love. It authenticates love, purifies its motives, and makes it more Christ-like. Indeed, the self-emptying love that is *necessary* for the raising of children is not only an imitation of Christ's self-offering, but a real participation in it. The procreation of children is an exercise of our common priesthood: like Christ, who offered himself as priest and victim, we offer ourselves as a gift to our spouse and children for their good *and* for ours. For by offering ourselves to others we learn who we really are: "Whoever finds his life will lose it, and whoever loses his life for my sake will find it" (Mt 10:39).

The Crucifix that hangs above the marriage bed of so many Catholic households takes on new meaning in this light. In the same way that the cross

---

[32] The blessing of this openness is available even to childless couples. "Spouses to whom God has not granted children can nevertheless have a conjugal life full of meaning, in both human and Christian terms. Their marriage can radiate a fruitfulness of charity, of hospitality, and of sacrifice." *Catechism of the Catholic Church* 1654

effected a self-emptying offering that literally produced children for God, the marriage bed effects a sharing in this once-for-all sacrifice to produce children for God. It is no mere metaphor that Christ refers to his Church as His bride and to Himself as the Bridegroom. On Holy Thursday, Christ proclaimed his marriage vows—"This is my body which will be given up for you"—and on Good Friday He consummated the marriage on the Cross. For this reason two of the Doctors of the Catholic Church, St. Teresa of Avila and Saint John of the Cross, likened the Cross to the marriage bed. Jesus formed a union with the people of God, He consummated it on the cross to bring forth divine progeny, and He appointed marriage as the sacramental sign of this marvelous offering (cf. Eph 5:25-32).

That the rearing of children engenders self-sacrificial love in parents is an essential element of the marriage vocation but children must be seen not only in their benefits to the marriage. On the contrary, a child is a supreme good in and of himself (cf. John Paul II *Letter to Families* No. 11). What gift is more precious than life itself? Into the marriage is sent a new person who did not exist before, an immortal soul created by God through an intimate expression of love between husband and wife. A child is the consummate instance of God's miraculous intervention in the lives of his people. How can we not welcome such a magnificent blessing? How can we refuse such a generous calling?

That children are the "supreme gift" of marriage and an essential element of marital love has been the subject of a number of Papal audiences from Pope John Paul II:

> God's blessing is at the origin not only of marital communion, but also of a responsible and generous openness to life. Children really are the "springtime of the family and society"…It is in children that marriage blossoms: they crown that total partnership of life which makes husband and wife "one flesh"; this is true both of the children born from the natural relationship of the spouses and those desired through adoption. Children are not an "accessory" to the project of married life. They are not an "option," but a "supreme gift," inscribed in the very structure of the conjugal union. The Church, as you know, teaches an ethic of respect for this fundamental structure in both its unitive and procreative meaning. In all this, it expresses the proper regard for God's plan, sketching an image of conjugal relations that are marked by mutual and unreserved acceptance. Above all, it addresses the right of children to be born and to grow in a context of fully human love. In conforming to the word of God, families thus become a school of humanization and true solidarity (*Sunday Homily, Jubilee of Families,* October 15, 2000).

In choosing marriage as our vocation, we accept, prospectively, the gift of children. In fact the vows taken in marriage require our assent to "accept children from God lovingly and bring them up according to the law of Christ and His Church." This is a sacred pledge to God and spouse before witnesses—a vow that if kept produces new life that quickens our will to love and enlivens our outlook. Pope John Paul II spoke poetically to this point in an October 14, 2000, address to families:

> Do not children themselves in a way continually "examine" their parents? They do so not only with their frequent "whys?", but with their very faces, sometimes smiling, sometimes misty with sadness. It is as if a question were inscribed in their whole existence, a question which is expressed in the most varied ways, even in their whims, and which we could put into questions like these: Mama, papa, do you love me? Am I really a gift to you? Do you accept me for what I am? Do you always try to do what is really best for me?
>
> These questions perhaps are asked more with their eyes than in words, but they hold parents to their great responsibility and are in some way an echo of God's voice for them.
>
> Children are a "springtime": what does this metaphor chosen for your Jubilee mean?
>
> It takes us into that panorama of life, colors, light, and song which belongs to the spring season. Children are all of this by nature. They are the hope that continually blossoms, a project that starts ever anew, the future that opens without ceasing. They represent the flowering of married love, which is found and strengthened in them. At their birth they bring a message of life, which, in the ultimate analysis, refers back to the very Author of life. In need of everything as they are especially in the first stage of life, they naturally appeal to our solidarity.
>
> Not by chance did Jesus invite his disciples to have a child's heart. Today, dear families, you wish to give thanks for the gift of children and, at the same time, to accept the message that God sends you through their existence (*Third World Meeting with Families*).

Jesus taught, "Let the children come to me and do not prevent them, for the kingdom of God belongs to such as these" (Lk. 18:16). Children are the model of a kingdom people. They are the living symbol of hope, innocence, and life itself. Indeed, Jesus came to us as a child, bearing in his infancy a new beginning for humanity. How fitting that our restoration would be revealed to us in the new life of a tender little baby. Every newborn child reminds us of our capacity for renewal and our unique ability to shape the future of God's kingdom.

Review Questions

1. How do the sacrifices parents make for children strengthen love of God and neighbor in parents?

2. In his October 15, 2000 Jubilee of Families homily, John Paul II teaches that conjugal union, "sketches an image of conjugal relations that are marked by" what?

3. What metaphor is Pope John Paul II describing when he says, "They are the hope that continually blossoms, a project that starts ever anew, the future that opens without ceasing"?

Discussion Question

How do you think children are the "springtime of the family and of society" (Jubilee of Families Homily, October 15, 2000)?

Chapter 9
Discerning "just" and "serious" reasons for postponing pregnancy

"Those are also considered to be responsible who, for serious reasons and with due respect for moral precepts, decide not to have another child for either a definite or an indefinite period of time."

> Pope Paul VI, *Humanae Vitae* 10

"Certainly there may be just reasons for spacing offspring: these may be based on the physical or psychological condition of the spouses, or may be based on external factors."

> *Humanae Vitae* 16

How should a couple discern "just" and "serious" reasons for postponing pregnancy?

Intentions and Motivation

Spouses are called to have children, as children are the "supreme good" of married life (CCC 1664). However, there is no obligation to have as many children as physically possible without consideration of circumstances. Rather, the Church teaches that procreation may be regulated under certain conditions:

> For *just* reasons, spouses may wish to space the births of their children. It is their duty to make certain that their desire is not motivated by selfishness but is in conformity with the generosity appropriate to responsible parenthood. Moreover, they should conform their behavior to the objective criteria of morality. (CCC 2368).
>
> Those are also to be considered responsible who for *serious* reasons [*seriis causis*] and with due respect for moral precepts, decide not to have another child for either a definite or an indefinite amount of time.[33]

The Church provides some guidelines for determining when it is moral to have children and when it is moral to postpone or cease having children. The decision must be considered in light of the Christian virtues of self-donation, charity, and prudence. Self-donation and charity, which are so closely related as to be practically synonymous, demand that the decision to have children consider first and foremost the good of the children (both existing and future), that is, a selfless appraisal of the intrinsic value of another child and his/her welfare. Prudence calls us to make wise and responsible decisions in service of charity and guides charity to its most fruitful end.

It is neither prudent nor charitable to have more children than a couple can reasonably care for. Indeed, Karol Wojtyla (John Paul II) teaches in his book *Love and Responsibility* that the prudent exercise of the gift of procreation is part of responsible parenthood:

> There are, however, circumstances in which this disposition [to be a responsible parent] itself demands renunciation of procreation, and any further increase in the size of the family would be

---

[33] HV 10, Trans: Janet Smith, see Additional Resources section p.143.

incompatible with parental duty. A man and a woman moved by true concern for the good of their family and a mutual sense of responsibility for the birth, maintenance, and upbringing of their children, will then limit intercourse and abstain from it in periods in which this might result in another pregnancy undesirable in the particular conditions of their married life and family.[34]

Specific Criteria

Humanae Vitae teaches that there are four factors that must be weighed in order to make a prudent decision to procreate: physical, psychological, economic, and social (HV 10). While there is no checklist of specific criteria formulated by the Church for these factors, we can reasonably identify the more obvious points. Danger to the physical well-being of the mother and/or child, inability to physically provide basic care for children, severe mental disability that makes responsible parenthood impossible—all of these could be serious or just reasons for postponing children. External factors might include an inability to provide for the basic needs of the children (e.g., food, shelter, clothing, safe environment, adequate education, medical care), serious marital instability, spousal abuse, gross lack of spousal support, and unemployment, to name a few.

These more obvious criteria may not describe the situation of many couples, in whose case the decision to procreate is a clearer calling and obligation though not without some degree of ambiguity and moral deliberation. In these cases it might be more helpful to identify what could be considered invalid or selfish motives for the postponement of children. Loss of free time, sense of lost youth, cramped social life, inconvenience, change in sex life, inopportune timing, distaste for baby's bodily functions (diaper changing, spit-up, slobber, crying, etc.), and materialism (inordinate attachment to material possessions), arguably all fall short of the standard of *just* or *serious* reasons.

The Second Vatican Council's *Pastoral Constitution on the Church in the Modern World* also offers some criteria for discerning the call to have children:

> Parents should regard as their proper mission the task of transmitting human life and educating those to whom it has been transmitted. They should realize that they are thereby cooperators with the love of God the Creator, and are, so to speak, the interpreters of that love. Thus they will fulfill their task with human and Christian responsibility, and, with docile reverence toward God, will make

---

[34] *Love and Responsibility.* Ignatius Press. San Francisco: 1993, p. 243.

decisions by common counsel and effort. Let them thoughtfully take into account both their own welfare and that of their children, those already born and those which the future may bring. For this accounting they need to reckon with both the material and the spiritual conditions of the times as well as of their state in life. Finally, they should consult the interests of the family group, of temporal society, and of the Church herself. The parents themselves and no one else should ultimately make this judgment in the sight of God. But in their manner of acting, spouses should be aware that they cannot proceed arbitrarily, but must always be governed according to a conscience dutifully conformed to the divine law itself, and should be submissive toward the Church's teaching office, which authentically interprets that law in the light of the Gospel. That divine law reveals and protects the integral meaning of conjugal love, and impels it toward a truly human fulfillment. Thus, trusting in divine Providence and refining the spirit of sacrifice, married Christians glorify the Creator and strive toward fulfillment in Christ when with a generous human and Christian sense of responsibility they acquit themselves of the duty to procreate. Among the couples who fulfill their God-given task in this way, those merit special mention who with a gallant heart, and with wise and common deliberation, undertake to bring up suitably even a relatively large family (GS 50).

The council urges that spouses balance the "duty" to procreate with their state in life, the welfare of their existing and future children, as well as the needs of the Church and the world. Their discernment should be imbued with the spirit of sacrifice and trust in divine providence. The concrete, practical living out of these ideals requires us to take stock of our priorities and consider what is really important in life. Our Lord taught, "seek first the kingdom of God and his justice, and all these things shall be given you besides" (Mt 6:33). Every good in our lives hinges on our relationship with God, whether the good is material means, personal fulfillment, or companionship. If we fail to embrace the call of God by rejecting the goods with which he has endowed marriage, the things that we try to put in place of these goods are emptied of their significance. Pitting our plans against God's can never lead to fulfillment. Trusting in God's providence in the spirit of sacrifice places our desires at the disposal of God with the confidence that He knows what is best for us and will never stop caring for us.

Getting Your Ducks in a Row

A serious decision of conscience such as this requires prayer—honest, deep, and persistent prayer. Guidance from priests, NFP couples, holy friends and family, books, tapes, and videos help provide direction and conscience formation. Cutting costs, living more simply, and reprioritizing our material desires, can help eliminate financial obstacles to choosing parenthood or a larger family. A couple should do everything they can to make a truly informed choice based on the objective norms for marriage and procreation revealed in the Church. In cases of doubt and indecision, the choice to postpone parenthood without consulting the teaching of the Church, without prayer and soul-searching, and without the advice of authorities, is remiss.

Because marriage, by its very nature, is ordered to the procreation and education of children (CCC 1652), spouses have a responsibility to steer their circumstances, over time, in the direction of having children. Excepting the rare cases of spouses who are physically, psychologically, economically, or socially *incapable* of caring for children, spouses are called to actively plan their lives for the eventuality of having children. Steps must be taken to facilitate openness to life in attitude and circumstance even if the couple has chosen to take some time to think about it. Couples who neglect these steps—prayer, inquiry, introspection, financial self-control—have never really entered the realm of conscientious deliberation but may have *a priori* closed themselves to new life.

Listening to Our Bodies

Natural Family Planning opens the door for couples to *listen to their bodies* in the discernment of whether to welcome or postpone children. The desire for the marital embrace should not be reduced to a purely physiological impulse. Rather, it should be understood as a divinely crafted inclination that harmonizes physical desire with actual grace (divine prompting toward some good). In other words, the sexual impulse toward our spouse is a means of Divine suggestion. If we are constantly and indefinitely denying attraction to our spouse, we may need to *consider* (prayerfully weigh the possibility in consultation with one's spouse) relaxing the rules for the postponement of children and take some chances, realizing that children are often a greater blessing than we can ever imagine.

Too often couples expect the will of God to manifest itself like a lightning bolt from heaven—infusing them with certain knowledge of God's will—while they ignore the more ordinary channels through which God communicates. God speaks to us through our sexuality, and these urges created by God also respond to His providential guidance. This is *not* to say that we are slaves to our natural impulses. As rational creatures, we cooperate intelligently with the creator in the choices we make. The presence and timing of attraction toward our spouse is not an automatic mandate from God that we must have children, but it should factor into our discernment of whether we will accept the vocation of parenthood, or the invitation to be open to another child.

Discerning the Call to Parenthood in the Larger Context of Faith

Like all moral decisions, the choice of whether to have a child is affected by the overall condition of our faith. The best way to prepare for such a life-changing decision is to (1) embrace the baptismal call to holiness in youth, (2) exercise sound judgment in choosing a spouse, (3) avoid premarital sex and cohabiting relationships in favor of loving and communicative relationships, and (4) develop the obedience of faith wherein we submit ourselves completely to the will of God.

Marriage preparation, seen in this light, begins in childhood. In fact, the Pontifical Council for the Family teaches that education in the meaning of marriage actually begins before birth in the atmosphere in which the new life is awaited and welcomed as a gift.[35] Parents, priests, and youth ministers are obliged to model obedience, chastity, prayer, and openness to new life across the various ministerial settings. Attitudes are formed in our youth that determine our receptiveness to the Church's teaching on contraception, NFP, and the blessings of children in our adult years. Those responsible for the formation of youth have a responsibility to actively structure the dating attitudes and practices of young people so they learn early the real meaning of love as mutual self-donation, not mutual gratification. This type of formation conforms our will to God's will, which remains always open to love and life. This more comprehensive approach will help eliminate the "loophole morality" that seeks the minimum number of children a couple is "required" to have and helps open marriages to the blessings of children and to the possibility of a large family. The fertility of marriage is not a numbers game but abandonment to God's plan of joyous spousal love and the flourishing of new life.

A Personal Note

New life is what this whole process of discernment is all about, although it gets obscured sometimes in our discernment of the legal/moral obligations of marriage and parenthood. In the end *life* is the weightiest of all the criteria for discerning the call to parenthood. After all, life is the good which parenthood serves. This was brought home to my wife and me in the birth of our first child. For all the soul searching, study, discussion, and anxiety that accompanied our decision to have children, nothing convinced us more that parenthood was God's call for us than when we embraced our

---

[35] *Preparation for the Sacrament of Marriage* 23

new little baby boy. Once he came into our lives, there was never a second thought about whether we had made the right decision.

We planned for the birth of our first child first by relaxing the rules of NFP for postponement of children. As we did this our openness to children increased, until eventually we began actively and intentionally using the fertile times to *achieve pregnancy*. I firmly believe that once we allowed God a glimmer of access to our wills, he infused us with the desire to have children. Time and time again we have found ourselves wondering what all the worry was about as we enjoy our life as parents. Even though we have never worked harder or sacrificed so much, we have never felt more fulfilled and we have never been happier. Our children are an unfathomable gift from God of which we feel unworthy.

Once I worried about what I would have to give up in having children; now I know there is nothing that I would not give up for my children. They are infinitely more valuable to me than anything I own. They have deepened my love for my wife, and they have improved the way I spend my time. I see that I am a better person now than before, and that my potential is more fully realized because of this gift. We may have less disposable income, but we have learned to live happily on less. Simpler living has revealed to us just how much money we used to waste; parenthood has made us better stewards.

The bottom line is that all of my concerns about having children were obliterated the moment our son was born. We now have two beautiful children and hope to have more. The future growth of our family is still a subject of much prayer and discussion, but with far less anxiety and trepidation, because we have learned firsthand just how blessed parenthood can be. We are living life to the fullest, entrusting our family and our future to God.

Some Final Words on Discerning Parenthood

The final word on discerning parenthood is that there is no final word on discerning parenthood. It is tempting to want or demand a definitive checklist for making a decision, a kind of flowchart that produces a quick and certain answer to a complex question. The Church is clear on the responsibility of spouses to remain open to children and to avoid illicit means of postponing them (i.e., contraception). But the application of these norms may be more fluid than we would like them to be. We like clear and simple answers to questions, but we are not going to find one here. While the call to marriage is by its nature a call to parenthood, the choice of when to begin having children or whether to have another child should be worked out in prayer, honest communication among spouses, and good counsel from holy people, in light of the Church's objective moral teachings on the goods of marriage and the conjugal union. There is pressure from both ends of the spectrum on this issue. Those with a so-called "contraceptive mentality," or worse, those who ignore the issue altogether, want to deny the marital call to parenthood entirely in complete rebellion toward the meaning of marriage and the teaching authority of the Church. Spouses who pursue children with the attitude that more is *always* better without considering the impact on their family often put pressure on others to pursue parenthood without discernment or forethought. Both of these views polarize and complicate the discernment process unnecessarily. There simply is no one-size-fits-all approach to this issue because no two marriages or families are the same. Objective norms can be taught and reiterated, reasonable parameters can be set to help guide the process by ruling out frivolous reasons for postponing children, and methods of facilitating openness to children can be suggested. But the interplay between the human conscience and the truth that binds it is too subtle and complex to neatly wrap up in one fell swoop.

To those who are frustrated with the lack of definition in the discernment process, consider this distinction. When the moral decision facing us involves the prohibition of an intrinsic evil, such as abortion, our choice is unambiguous—we may never commit abortion under any circumstances. If we, by a positive act of the will, commit an action that is intrinsically evil, we have done wrong. When the moral decision facing us involves whether, or to what extent, we are to perform some positive good, the choice is less clear. For example, going to Mass is a morally good choice to which I am obligated every Lord's Day. Does it then follow that I decide against this good [the Mass] if I don't go every day? Is it the case that if it is good to go to Mass, then I have sinned against this good if I don't go at every given opportunity? It is good, moreover, to adore the Blessed Sacrament because it is the Real Presence of Christ. Have I done wrong, if knowing this, I don't spend every waking moment in front of the Tabernacle in prayer?

Apply these scenarios to the discernment of parenthood. The choice to contracept is an intrinsically evil act, the willful commission of a prohibited deed, and is therefore clearly wrong. When our choice is whether to have children, when to have them, or whether to have more, it is not a matter of prohibition but of the commission of a good deed. Children are intrinsically good, but does this mean that if I don't have as many as possible I am sinning against this good? I am not obligated to have as many children as physically possible any more than I am obligated to attend Mass or to visit the Blessed Sacrament as many times as physically possible. The standard that I must follow in deciding to promote these goods is generosity—giving all I can to promote a good *prudently*. You can see how this standard would be different for different people in different states of life. This is where the fluidity of discerning parenthood is revealed. Like the commission of any other good, we must determine our obligations insofar as they serve the good we want to promote.[36] Getting involved in parish ministries, for example, is good; but it ceases to be good if in doing so I neglect my children, my wife, and the career with which I support them. Likewise, having children is good, but if we have more than we can support, we endanger the welfare of all our children and compromise the stability of our marriage. The *generous* approach is, in the former example, to involve myself in parish ministry as much as I can without compromising my family and career. In the latter example, I am generous when I have as many children as I can without compromising the welfare of my existing children and the stability of my marriage.[37]

Keeping Our Objectivity

It is wise at this point to reiterate that we must always abide by the objective teaching of the Church that children are a natural end of marriage and that the conjugal act must always remain open to new life. This is why the Church upholds the standard of *serious* or *just* reasons for the postponement of procreation. In the absence of these reasons it is understood that couples would not try to limit their acts of intercourse to the infertile periods. That the choice to not impede having children takes into consideration certain circumstances does not make it a purely subjective matter—the couple must make their choice within the bounds of the Church's authoritative teaching.

It is our duty to apply the objective standards of married life to our discernment of parenthood to the best of our ability, utilizing (1) input from authorities loyal to the teaching of the Church, (2) our prayer life, (3) the grace of the sacraments, and (4) communication between spouses. Availing ourselves of all of these resources maximizes God's input on the matter, which is what will ultimately give us the answers we seek. We will be spared a lot of anxiety if we remind ourselves that God knows we are not infallible, and he does not expect an infallible decision from us on this matter. God does not say to us, "I will cooperate with you to bring about new life, but if you get it wrong I will smite you!" God's will is solicitous more than it is demanding. Of course, his will is certain and immutable but he brings us to his will as a teacher and loving father. It seems inconsistent with the

---

[36] See chapter 4 "Bishops Speak" for a treatment of the relationship between conscience and objective moral norms. See also *Veritatis Splendor* 59.

[37] See *Veritatis Splendor* 52 for further discussion of moral prohibitions versus the obligation to do good.

nature of God that he would want us to be fearful or anxious over the decision to have children. On the contrary, it seems more likely that God would like us to see the decision to have children the same way we might see a decision about who we will marry—exciting, full of expectation, hopeful, and passionate. The only way our discernment of parenthood will be these things to us is if we love our spouse generously and allow God into the discernment process in every way possible.

It follows that family life ministers and/or other teachers of the Church's vision for marriage and family life explain not only the harm of contraception and the blessings of children, but that they offer couples friendly guidance about whether, when, and how large to make a family. It is not fair or wise to offer teaching in the methodology of NFP during marriage preparation and then to forget about these couples. NFP is an essential part of marriage preparation and follow-up is equally essential—it is more than a method; it is a ministry that is ongoing. Dioceses/parishes ought to provide open-ended support and direction for couples trying to decide whether they want to begin or expand families. Parishes should conduct workshops, retreats, and days of recollection that specifically address this issue, wherein couples learn the Church's wisdom on the issue and are given a variety of opportunities to examine themselves:

1. Meetings with seasoned parents who can articulate their experience with the discernment process and their experience as parents;

2. Time alone to discuss with each other where they are on the issue of openness to children;

3. Instruction on financial considerations—living more simply and avoiding materialism;

4. Explanation of how to make prayer part of the decision-making process;

5. Discussion of appropriate and inappropriate criteria for postponing children;

6. Offering a Parenthood Support Group in the parish that will help couples who have decided to pursue achieving pregnancy.

Conducting events like these is easier than it might seem. NFP couples are usually more than willing and capable to help with this type of project—all it would take is a few motivated couples to make it work.

Couples who know they have the support of friends are much less anxious about the prospect of having children. Making a big decision alone is scary, but is less frightening when made with the help of trusted advisors. Parishioners will be much more open to children if they feel they don't have to go it alone. When the parish is seen by married couples as a support network that will welcome and nurture their children—as well as provide a helping hand in their upbringing and formation—they will be encouraged to begin or expand their families. Yet parents are not the only ones to benefit from this kind of support. Vibrant, loving families are a wellspring of renewal for the parish and the whole Church. It is hard not to notice that parishes with an atmosphere of vitality and enthusiasm, parishes that are growing and reaching out to others, are full of robust families. We can see that the parish community is an essential partner in the discernment process of spouses, providing guidance, practical support, and an environment in which the gifts of the family bear fruit for the family of God at large.

Review Questions

1. The Catechism of the Catholic Church (2368) teaches that couples wishing to space the births of their children should conform their behavior to what?

2. *Humanae Vitae* (10) teaches that there are four criteria for judging "just" and "serious" reasons for postponing children; what are they?

3. What are some examples of possible external factors that may justify postponing children?

4. What four steps should be taken to guide the discernment process to have children (or more children) or to postpone them?

Discussion Question

In general, there seems to be a threefold spectrum of positions with regard to moral guidelines for responsible procreation:

> (1) **The Contraceptive Mentality,** which holds that fertility is to be hindered by direct and willful measures to separate the unitive and procreative elements of conjugal acts. It is comprised primarily of the use of contraception: chemical, prophylactic, surgical, withdrawal, or abortifacient. The contraceptive mentality occurs in a different way, however, in the use of a natural method of family planning that is in-

definitely or permanently closed to new life for unjust or non-serious reasons. This second instance is harder to identify because it is less direct than contraception.

(2) **Natural Family Planning** used for just and serious reasons discerned by thorough examination of conscience, prayer, advice of authorities, discussion, and trust in God's providence.

(3) **"Providentialism,"** which holds that no means of fertility management are desirable and that NFP undermines God's plan for the fecundity of marriage. Advocates maintain that there should be no method for postponing pregnancy that involves the conscious and deliberate postponement of pregnancy.

The question is in two parts:

(A) Is this a fair categorization of the spectrum of positions regarding responsible procreation?

(B) What are the merits of these positions?

Part II
Pastoral Considerations

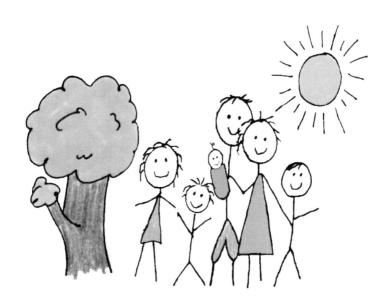

How faith communities can create an NFP culture liberated from contraception and open to the blessings of children

❶ Include a full course of NFP in marriage preparation programs.

Parish leadership—pastors, DREs, parish coordinators, and catechists—must accept the *need* for NFP formation in the parish. In fact, the United States Conference of Catholic Bishops has instructed dioceses to include Natural Family Planning in their marriage preparation programs: *"We urge that premarriage programs require a full course of instruction in Natural Family Planning as a necessary component in the couple's effective realization of what they need and have a right to know in order to live in accord with the clear teaching of the Church."*[38] Once it is established that the Church forbids the use of contraception and sterilization for family planning, a teaching with which couples in marriage preparation should be keenly familiar, positive alternatives must be provided. If not, couples who are unaware of natural methods, or confuse them with outmoded methods will consider the Church's teaching burdensome, irrelevant and unreasonable.

A full course of NFP instruction, which includes a complete presentation of the moral, methodological, and scientific/physiological aspects of NFP, will equip couples to embrace the Church's teaching on marital sexuality and contraception with greater ease. Moreover, a full course in NFP will inculcate not just a methodology but a *way of life* that is open to the gift of fertility, total reciprocal self-giving, and the blessings of children. Natural Family Planning is hence an integral part of marriage preparation in that it requires openness, communication, selflessness, discipline, and commitment—all of which are prerequisites to a valid and successful marriage. NFP instruction, when seen in this light, fits marital preparation seamlessly, supporting the couples' formation in all varieties of marital "intercourse": physical, mental, spiritual, and emotional.

❷ Introduce Natural Family Planning to adult converts in RCIA programs.

Parish leaders must be sensitive to the fact that many inquirers in RCIA are engaged couples in which one or both partners are seeking marriage in the

---

[38] United States Conference of Catholic Bishops (USCCB), *Faithful to Each Other Forever: A Catholic Handbook of Pastoral Help for Marriage Preparation*, 1988, p. 47.

Church but are not yet Catholic. A *full course* in NFP is not necessarily appropriate in this setting, but a survey of the main tenets and an introduction to the methodology could be devised simply. Guest speakers (NFP teaching couples, nurses or doctors trained in NFP, diocesan NFP and/or Family Life Coordinators) are a good resource for a brief one or two class introduction. Needless to say, it is imperative that RCIA team members fully embrace the Church's teaching on contraception and the blessings of children—a unified catechesis is essential.

For many couples, initial exposure to NFP instruction produces tentative curiosity more than an instant conversion. For this reason, it is advisable to provide couples with materials they can take home and review: books, pamphlets, tapes, videos, websites, and phone numbers for further information. Couples should also be given contact information for NFP couples who are willing to discuss NFP, which brings us to our next tool.

❸ Assemble a team of NFP-using couples who are willing to give testimonials and counsel with engaged and married couples.

The testimony of couples who have successfully incorporated NFP into their marriages and who can speak to its advantages are perhaps the most effective means of persuading engaged and married couples to explore Natural Family Planning. Testimonial/Consultant couples personalize the Church's case for natural methods, and provide needed support and advice for inquiring couples. Panel testimonies in which several couples of varying ages and states in life provide testimony to parishioners about the benefits of NFP are an indispensable part of couples' formation. If testimonial couples are willing to make a deeper commitment, they can ease into the role of consultants, making themselves available for phone consultation, or opening their homes for a visit from couples who want to know more. This kind of openness and personal attention surpasses didactic instruction and actually *disciples* couples into the NFP lifestyle.

While engaged couples seeking marriage in the Church are especially suited to NFP instruction, there are many couples in the parish *already married* that have not chosen NFP. The parish family must not turn a blind eye to these latter couples, who are equally in need of instruction and discipleship. Testimonial evenings can be organized apart from marriage preparation classes in special events like dinners and even outings, which offer a non-threatening fellowship. Dinners and outings create a friendly, casual environment in which NFP couples and non-NFP couples blend, as opposed to an instructional setting in which inquirers assume a student status, implying that they are non-NFP couples. Anonymity, at least initially, can be a comfort to the curious.

❹ **Equip families to instruct their children in the Church's teaching on contraception and the blessings of children.**

The Church refers to the family as the "Domestic Church" because it is the first and most influential faith formation a person receives. Especially pertinent to catechesis in marital relations, it is the first school of human interaction and relationships. Instruction in NFP begins, not with sex, but with the example of parents, who by their interaction with each other and their children, model openness to life, self-sacrificial love, and obedience to the natural law. Put simply, children learn from their parents that Natural Family Planning fosters a happier marriage.

Parish adult education programs should accordingly address the Church's vision for sexuality in marriage and NFP. Such instruction should be broadly integrated into Bible studies, courses for *parents seeking baptism for their children*, married and engaged encounters, retreats, parish missions, seasonal programs like Lenten series and observances of feasts, pro-life initiatives, and social justice campaigns. It is not necessary to invent a lot of new NFP-centered programs. Existing programs can be supplemented to include NFP and its corollaries. This is perhaps more desirable as it communicates to the parish that NFP is part and parcel of not just the vocation of marriage, but the vocation to holiness to which we are all called.

❺ **Preach NFP from the pulpit.**

Catechesis for most adult Catholics occurs during the homily of Sunday Mass. The homily is the primary instance of formal public instruction in human sexuality and beginning of life issues, *including contraception and NFP*. Pastors are charged with the duty of fathering their congregation away from bondage to sin and toward freedom in the truth: "If you remain in my word, you will truly be my disciples, and you will know the truth, and the truth will set you free" (Jn 8:32). Whereas the use of contraception is a significant obstacle to Christian freedom, fulfillment, and happiness, Natural Family Planning is a gateway to these goals in marriage. In general, NFP marriages enjoy greater freedom, fulfillment, and happiness which is evidenced in their almost non-existent divorce rate. In an age of throwaway marriages, couples should be given from every source possible a pathway to a joyful, successful marriage. What pastor would not desire this for his children: "What father among you would hand his son a snake when he asks for a fish? Or hand him a scorpion when he asks for an egg?" (Lk 11:11,12)?

Can preaching NFP help solve a shortage of vocations to priesthood?

Preaching NFP is not only beneficial to parishioners, but also to the clergy. We ought to ask ourselves what effect, if any, contraception has had on the apparent lack of new vocations to the priesthood. The median age of priests is increasing, and so is their workload. Clergy are often asked to pastor two or three parishes concurrently, working from early morning to late evening fulfilling their sacramental and organizational duties, pressured to oversee all sorts of parish and diocesan initiatives, all the while trying to maintain an interior life. While priests do a laudable job at balancing these demands, both clergy and laity could benefit from an influx of new priests. We must consider the possibility that smaller families, resulting largely from a contraceptive culture, are less likely to produce young men for the priesthood. Social customs influence parents to desire the propagation of the family name through their sons, and parents naturally desire grandchildren. While neither of these concerns is trivial, both are logically intensified when there are fewer children in the family. Parents might tend to be "freer" with their children if they have more of them.

There are two common objections to preaching NFP: (1) parishioners will object to the message and vote against it, as it were, with their feet; and (2) direct instruction on NFP neglects the readings, from which the homily is supposed to proceed. That parishioners will object to the message is insufficient reason to conceal the truth. This part of the truth is one our married couples desperately need, and the love of Christ compels us. Recall the many times Jesus preached a message that was unpopular to his public, or how many times prophets and martyrs like John the Baptist stuck their necks out for the truth. Yet, neither Jesus nor John the Baptist had any shortage of disciples. Compassion demands the truth, especially when so much is riding on it. Without a clear understanding of contraception and NFP many otherwise sound marriages will fail with incalculable damage to the spouses, the children, and the community. We must not let fear of rejection cause us to allow members of our community to continue on a destructive path.

The growth and appeal of Christianity throughout the ages has been the result of an uncompromising proclamation of the truth. What have we to fear, furthermore, when we have been granted the Spirit of truth through whom the Apostle Peter converted three thousand with a message that was forbidden by authorities? In his last instructions to the Apostles, through whom Holy Orders has descended to the priesthood, Christ commissioned the Apostles to teach *all* that He had commanded. Saint Paul, accepting this mandate fully, declared, "If I preach the gospel, this is no reason for me to boast, *for an obligation has been imposed on me, and woe to me if I do not preach it!"* (1 Cor 9:16). The obligation here is love—willing the good of another. Simple love for the married members and the families of our communities will drive us to give them the tools they need to succeed.

Courage in preaching the Gospel is easy to discuss in the abstract but in the "real world" of parish life and politics, can it be done? Aside from the fact that the Gospel has always been preached in the *real world*, sometimes at great sacrifice, courageous emphasis on NFP has proven rewarding for many priests. Father Randall Moreau, of the Diocese of Lafayette, Louisiana, claims that a growing NFP culture in his parish has enlivened volunteerism and lightened his workload:

> Natural family planners make great volunteers…willing to make sacrifices for the Church, for God, for us priests, constantly. "NFPers" far outdo the average volunteers…and for so much longer than the average volunteer. [They] are passionate about our work, the salvation of souls…because they want souls; because they know…that what is at stake is souls. They know it's not just the priest's job to save souls, it's everybody's job... (CD presentation "Why NFP is a Priority in My Parish" available from One More Soul, individually and as part of a 3 CD set "NFP Talks for Clergy" see p. 144)

Greater openness to God's providence in the area of marital sexuality can be seen in two ways, either as a gateway to greater openness in other areas of spirituality and morality, or as the removal of a last hindrance to complete abandonment to Christ. Some would say that in the former case, the giving over to God of our sexuality initiates a pattern of self-denial that stimulates other virtues. In the latter case, it may well be that we let loose a flood of virtue that has been constricted by our ignorance and/or recalcitrance on this issue. In either case, when the community entrusts its marriages and its outlook on human sexuality fully to God, it sets itself on a course of *advanced spirituality*. This pays dividends to diocesan parishes and schools. As a result, it is improbable, if not impossible, to find a priest who regrets creating a pro-fertility, pro-Natural Family Planning parish.

Father Frank Pavone, president of *Priests for Life*, testifies to the positive effects of making NFP central to parish ministry for engaged couples:

> Is it possible for a parish in the United States today to require the couples who get married there to learn NFP? Not only is it possible, but it is happening, right in New York City.
>
> After my ordination in 1988, I was appointed parochial vicar at St. Charles parish, in the Oakwood Heights section of Staten Island. St. Charles registers about 3600 families, mostly of Irish and Italian descent. It has an average number of 68 weddings a year.
>
> If a couple wishes to be married at St. Charles, they are required to take a course in Natural Family Planning. This has been a parish policy for about fifteen years. The course, which is in addition to the usual Pre-Cana and meetings with the priest, is offered at a local Catholic hospital, St. Vincent's, and consists in three evening sessions. (Since the third session is designed for those who have already begun using the method, the engaged couples take only the first two sessions.)
>
> What's the reaction? Overwhelmingly, the couples appreciate having taken the sessions. Initially, there is sometimes a question as to why they need to do this when "my friend did not have to when she got married in her parish." We explain to them that we are committed to giving them the best possible preparation, so that they will be as fully equipped as possible to live a Catholic marriage. We show them that we have *their* best interests at heart. We explain that we don't want them to ever feel they are in a dilemma of having to choose between planning their family and being a good Catholic.
>
> Follow-up is important. We ask them to bring us the certificate indicating they have attended Sessions I and II of the NFP course. Then we ask for feedback. Some of the reactions I've received are, "It was interesting—I never knew about those things before!" "There were a lot of charts, but as I listened I realized how useful it is." "At first we didn't see why we should go, but now I see the value of it. Every couple should know about this!"
>
> During all the years of this policy, we can only recall one couple who decided to go to another parish rather than have to take the NFP class.
>
> Yes, it is possible to spread the good news of NFP. We need to be willing to be real Shepherds, leading the way courageously, ready to eagerly point to NFP and say, "Look at this! This is

important—indeed, necessary—for you to know! This will bless your marriage." Ultimately, from the couples we lead in this way, there can only be one wise response: "Thank you!"[39]

The second objection, that the readings of the Mass are not geared to homilies on contraception and the blessings of children, underestimates the unfathomable depth of the Scriptures and the lessons they contain for an endless variety of moral questions. A word for word condemnation of contraception or the blessings of children need not appear in the readings for us to glean important lessons about openness to fertility, abandonment to providence, and the evils of sexual immorality. The Liturgy of the Word, moreover, is celebrated within the context of the liturgical year—seasons and feasts that provide a thematic backdrop to the readings. Many of these seasons and feasts contain important lessons for the proper ordering of marital love. The table on the following pages relates the readings of the Mass and the liturgical calendar to the Church's teaching on contraception and openness to children, in order to facilitate the planning of homilies on these subjects.

Opportunities for an NFP Homily

1. Seasonal Readings such as Advent, Christmas, Lent, and Easter:

Advent and Christmas

Advent and Christmas both contain readings in which the plan of God rests on the abandonment of his chosen ones to divine providence and their openness to life/children. The *fiat* of Mary in the annunciation—and to a lesser extent, that of Elizabeth—exemplify the unfolding of God's plan through the parents' openness to children. How many of us could rule out the possibility that a prophet might be born to us, someone who will help heal the world in extraordinary ways? How would the world have been different if Mary and Elizabeth, or Abraham and Sarah, or Adam and Eve had not accepted God's invitation to children? What would have become of the poor and indigent people of Calcutta if Mother Teresa's parents had refused their gift of fertility?

Easter

The Easter Season is all about new life and rebirth. Easter reveals to us a new humanity definitively redeemed—children of God and heirs to

---

[39] "Teaching NFP: A Step Forward," Fr. Frank Pavone, www.priestsforlife.org/articles/teachingnfp.html.

God's eternal life. Christ's resurrection is the consummate sharing of life, the transference of humanity from the state of servitude to the state of "children of God" (Rom 8:14-17). The Resurrection elevates humanity to *divine filiation*, that is, it makes us children of God and brothers and sisters in Christ. There is, perhaps, no better catechesis on the value and nature of childhood, therefore, than the Easter mystery, for children are the fruit of love. In the same way that our spiritual childhood is the fruit of Christ's love for His bride, the Church, children are the visible fruit of marriage. Love is always life giving and fruitful. This is why Christ's offering of love on the Cross did not end in death but in glorified life. If marriage is the visible sign of Christ's laying down His life for the Church (Eph 5:25-32), then it, too, must be oriented to giving life.

Trinitarian communion was revealed in the glorification of the Son in the Resurrection. The Resurrection is the sign, *par excellence*, of the life-giving power of God. The family, reflecting the Trinity, is a communion of persons that more effectively witnesses to God when it, too, gives life. Christ's resurrection applies God's life-giving power to humanity, creating the family of God. We, in turn, imitate, or rather, participate in this act when by our transmission of life, we create a family.

The family motif is carried on in **The Feast of the Ascension**, which anticipates our coming of age as children of God, and our consequent reception of the inheritance of the Father, the beatific vision. **Trinity Sunday** would likewise pertain to the Trinitarian significance of procreation and family as well as **The Feast of Pentecost**, because, just as children proceed from the mutual love of parents, the Holy Spirit proceeds as the personification of the mutual love of the Divine Persons. Our human relationships (communion among persons) naturally reflect the essence of God written into the creation. All creation bears the mark of its creator.

Preaching on NFP during Christmas and Easter has the added advantage of reaching Catholics who might not attend Mass regularly, but come out for special feasts. Pastors and parishioners alike are well aware of how much pew count swells during these two holy days. It may well be that this group of parishioners is the one most in need of catechesis on fertility and NFP, and what a brilliant opportunity to lend significance and solemnity to the message.

Lent

Lent is a time to accept our call to examine our consciences and repent from sin. Advent, too, with its emphasis on judgment and the bold preaching of John the Baptist to repentance in preparation for the coming of Christ, is a time to clean house spiritually. We must be ready to admit that, in light of the scandalously high number of Catholics who practice contraception and sterilization, we have distorted God's design for marital sexuality. Since Lent and Advent emphasize new beginnings, both might be occasions to introduce the subject of sterilization reversal, a real possibility for most sterilized couples (*see resources section for information on sterilization reversal*).

2. Prominent Feasts/Solemnities

Presentation of the Lord (Feb. 2)—Jesus is portrayed by the prophet Simeon as a sign that will be opposed, a sign of contradiction. Jesus is the quintessential symbol of standing against the prevailing sentiment of the age, of rising up against bondage to sin and error without counting the cost. The Presentation of the Lord, traditionally associated with the virtue of obedience so well modeled by Joseph and Mary's keeping of the Law, is well suited to the message that Christ has designed marriage to be fruitful despite the contraceptive mentality that so characterizes modern culture. We see in this feast a twofold offensive against a sinful culture: (1) Mary and Joseph's acceptance of a mission that would require radical self-denial, and (2) an instance of parents redeeming the culture surrendering their parenthood to divine providence. Generous openness to children in marriage is an exercise in both of these virtues. Accepting parenthood can change the world; Mary and Joseph are a testament to that.

St. Joseph, Husband of Mary (Mar. 19)—Husbands are often a stumbling block to the use of NFP in marriages. Saint Joseph cooperated with Mary's call to parenthood, accepting God's will with complete docility. Husbands must guard the purity of their wives, just as St. Joseph guarded Mary's purity. Joseph admirably fulfills the ideal established by St. Paul in his letter to the Ephesians: "Husbands, love your wives, even as Christ loved the Church and handed himself over for her to sanctify her, cleansing her by the bath of water with the word, that he might present to himself the Church in splendor, without spot or wrinkle or any such thing, that she might be holy and without blemish" (5:25-27). Husbands should not allow the purity and holiness of their wives to be compromised by supporting or coercing the use of contraception. This goes for sterilization as well, even to the male, for both spouses hereby participate in an act of coition that has been sterilized.

The Immaculate Conception (Dec. 8), The Annunciation (Mar. 25) & The Assumption (Aug. 15)—Mary, along with Abraham, is held up by the Church as an exemplar of the obedience of faith (CCC 148). Her will was wholeheartedly aligned with God's will, that is, she willed only what God willed, consenting even to the death of her beloved son, a horror spared Abraham. Disobedience to the plan of God was foreign to Mary, who surrendered her maternal rights in order to give her son as a sheep to slaughter. Likewise, disobedience to God's design for marriage, and the teaching of the Church He commissioned as our shepherd, should be equally foreign to us. Dissent was not an issue for Mary—she did not pursue loopholes; she was not concerned with whether Christ's will for her life was infallible or not—she gave herself without reservation because she loved Him truly: "Behold, I am the handmaid of the Lord" (The Annunciation, Lk 1:38). Thanks be to God for such love that brought us eternal redemption. Rebellion against the Church's clear and unwavering teaching on contraception, and the attendant desire of this rebellion to dominate and subvert our fertility, opposes the very archetype of redeemed humanity and deprives us of the divine life realized in her Assumption.

The Birth of John the Baptist (June 24)—John the Baptist is known for his passionate and hard-hitting preaching in preparation for the New Covenant. He called the world to repentance, urging it to make way for the Christ by making amends for its wrongdoing. His life was devoted to the circumcision of the heart (cf. Rm. 2:29) that would universalize salvation, making it possible for anyone, Jew or gentile, to be justified. His death came about as the result of his public condemnation of Herod's unlawful marriage to his brother's wife. The issue over which John gave up his life was the sanctity and right ordering of marriage. Can we not call ourselves to account for the disordering of marriage in our use of contraception and in our self-mutilative practice of sterilization? John the Baptist was no wild man, but a man of extraordinary conviction who deeply loved his people. His challenge, like that of the Church, is to clear the way for Christ by removing obstacles to full reception of His grace. Contraception is such an obstacle and until it is removed we cannot fully receive the gifts with which Christ has endowed marriage.

Saints Peter and Paul (June 29)—Out of the heroic sacrifice of saints Peter and Paul emerges a confirmation of the Christological ethic of leadership and service. Like Jesus before them, Peter and Paul laid down their lives to lead the Church, validating their commission as Apostolic fathers. Though this leadership exists today in the successors of the Apostles, rank and file Catholics too commonly dismiss Apostolic Succession by disobeying the teaching authority of the magisterium. Dissent from the Church's teaching on contraception, because this teaching has been the clear and continuous exercise of the apostolic office that resides in the Pope and the College of Bishops, is an implicit repudiation of the apostolicity of the Church. To reject the teaching authority of the Church on this matter is to reject the apostolic office sustained by Peter and Paul at so great a cost.

Body and Blood; Triumph of the Cross (Sept. 14)—Although we may not be proficient in the theology of redemptive suffering, most of us are familiar with the expression, "offer it up." Most of us are vaguely cognizant of the value of suffering for ourselves and others, though we do not like to suffer. The Triumph of the Cross opens up for us the mystery that our suffering can be united to that of Christ, not in such a way that Christ's offering on the Cross was insufficient and needs to be supplemented by our own suffering. Rather, it teaches us that our suffering is made efficacious because it is a participation in Christ's suffering: "Beloved, do not be surprised at the fiery ordeal which comes upon you to prove you, as though something strange were happening to you. But rejoice in so far as you share Christ's sufferings, that you may also rejoice and be glad when his glory is revealed" (1 Pt 4:12-13). Indeed, because Christ took upon Himself all human affliction on the Cross, he has already realized our suffering and offered it to God.

Our suffering has been, as it were, nailed to the Cross. Our personal self-sacrifices become one with Christ's self-sacrifice. We express this connection in the Mass during the offertory when we say, "May the Lord accept this sacrifice at your hands, for the praise and glory of God, for our good and the good of all of His Church." This shared sacrifice is redemptive to us *and to the rest of the Church* ("for our good and the good of all His Church"). Jesus does not offer Himself apart from us, exclusively. On the contrary, He offers Himself in union with humanity, incorporating us into His once-for-all sacrifice. He is our *corporate* representative, allowing all of the merit he earned to be applied to us, not juridically as if God simply demanded a pound of flesh for the wrongdoing of humanity, but communally, drawing his brothers and sisters (us) into an offering of love. Our every trial and our every act of love has meaning to the extent that it proceeds from the self-offering of Christ.

So what does this all have to do with contraception? We live in a hedonistic culture that tells us to pursue only what feels good, and to avoid all that feels bad by any means necessary. Parenthood and children have been assailed by this self-serving ethic. In the pursuit of sexual pleasure, material gain, and personal gratification, contraception has become the means of thwarting our fertility. Children are perceived by too many as an inconvenience—too costly, too time consuming, too needy. Yet, in keeping with the tenet that pleasure must be pursued at all costs, hedonism is not willing to let go of the sexual act that is designed to produce children. Modern culture is practically obsessed with the refinement of methods and gadgets that could "liberate" our sexuality from the threat and demands of parenthood. The result has been the objectification of persons: the turning of human beings into objects of sexual gratification. Love, which is the foundation and goal of romantic interaction, is replaced by infatuation and lust, creating counterfeit relationships that often end in separation and divorce.

Contraception, because it is aimed at mutual self-gratification instead of mutual self-gift, fuels this decline. Couples are trained to say with their bodies, "I give my whole self to you," while in truth withholding part of themselves from their partners. Standing against this degradation is the Triumph of the Cross, in which Jesus' heart matched perfectly His action. When He said, "This is my body given up for you," he enacted this promise bodily on the Cross. In His sacrifice is the very definition of love: the complete offering of self in recognition and service of another's God-given dignity. Jesus put the definition more simply: "No one has greater love than this, to lay down one's life for one's friends" (Jn 15:13).

Holy Family—What feast could be more suited to the message of the blessings of children and the harm of contraception? Mary and Joseph, despite the most difficult of circumstances, devoted themselves to the Christ child. Their openness to life was not hindered by the inconvenience of God's call for them, nor by the interruption of their plans for the future. Unlike the contracepting couple that says "no" to God's call to parenthood, Mary and Joseph said "yes." The faithfulness of the Holy Family in service to life, brought life to us all in the person of Christ. In the same way that Mary and Joseph found themselves in the vocation of parenthood, so too do we discover ourselves in our acceptance of this holy calling. The marriage of Joseph and Mary reveals to us that the raising of a child enhances the love of spouses for one another and deepens their shared sense of meaning to life. Theirs is a shining example of a sentiment common among parents: "It's the hardest thing I've ever done, but it's worth it!"

3. Anniversaries/Commemorations

Anniversary of Humanae Vitae (July 25)—Pope Paul VI's Encyclical *Humanae Vitae* is a concise summation of the Church's teaching on contraception. It defines the duties and responsibilities of conjugal love, the unitive and procreative aspects of sex, the morally impermissible methods of regulating birth, the morality of Natural Family Planning, and the consequences of artificial birth control for the world. There are, in fact, three consequences outlined by Pope Paul VI that have unfortunately been confirmed: (1) marital infidelity, (2) a general decline in morality, and (3) the abuse of contraceptive methods by public authorities. The high divorce rates we have experienced, the scandalous rate of out-of-wedlock pregnancies and fatherless families, and the coercive contraception and abortion policies that have emerged around the globe all prove *Humanae Vitae* right. The encyclical goes on to explain pastoral directives that emphasize self-mastery, and the creation of a climate of chastity. Appeals are made to public authorities, scientists, spouses, medical personnel, priests, and bishops, to uphold the truth about contraception and support openness to the blessings of children. It is a timeless document that, contrary to popular misconception, did not invent a new doctrine on fertility in marriage, but reiterated and clarified what the Church had always and universally taught.

Anniversary of Roe v. Wade (Jan. 22) & Respect Life Sunday (first Sun. in Oct.)

—Since 1973, nearly 42 million babies have been killed in the U.S.—a rate of approximately 1.5 million every year. While there is widespread agreement among Christians that abortion is an evil that must be eradicated (though agreement is not universal), there is much less awareness and agreement that contraception has fuelled the demand for abortion. Beyond the fact that the birth control pill is an abortifacient, contraception is based on intolerance of new life. Contraception assumes that fertility is a disease of sorts that must be treated with medication and which must be avoided by the use of prophylactics. The belief that we can artificially sterilize sex acts so as to avoid children implies a lack of appreciation for their value and opens the floodgates for a spectrum of other artificial measures that seek to achieve the same end through similarly illicit means. When we accept the use of contraception, we play into the hands of those who conspire against life: "It may be that many people use contraception with a view to excluding the subsequent temptation of abortion. But the negative values inherent in the 'contraceptive mentality'—which is very different from responsible parenthood, lived in respect for the full truth of the conjugal act—are such that they in fact strengthen this temptation when an unwanted life is conceived. Indeed, the pro-abortion culture is especially strong precisely where the Church's teaching on contraception is rejected" (EV 13). For this reason Pope John Paul II has described contraception and abortion as "fruits of the same tree" (EV 13). In an audience with the Austrian bishops, June 19, 1987 he was equally direct: "It is ever more clear that it is absurd, for instance, to want to overcome abortion through the promotion of contraception. The invitation to contraception as a supposedly 'harmless' manner of the relation between the sexes is not only an insidious denial of man's moral freedom. It fosters a depersonalized understanding of sexuality which is directed merely to the moment and promotes in the last analysis that mentality out of which abortion arises and from which it is continuously nourished. Furthermore, it is certainly not unknown to you that in more recent methods the transition from contraception to abortion has become extremely easy" (*L'Osservatore Romano*, July 13, 1987).

❻ **Organize conferences, missions, and retreats on NFP on a regular basis.**

Programs such as these should situate instruction on NFP and contraception within their parent topics, marriage and family and should characterize NFP as more than a method of family planning, but a *way of life* built on self-giving and obedience. Drawing upon the experience of married couples, and the expertise of clergy, moral theologians, and medical personnel, these special settings are an opportunity to "wake parishioners up," and reestablish the significance of NFP for married life. Many couples erroneously view the issue as passe, irrelevant, and idealistic. Put simply, they have moved on with their lives, suppressing any consideration of the morality of their approach to family planning. Conferences, missions, and retreats are opportunities for couples to stop and look around, to begin an examination of conscience with regard to their sexuality.

The parish is responsible for the *ongoing* education of adults in marital chastity, bringing to spouses a thorough understanding of the *whole* panoply of the marital embrace. This requires more than a one-time exposure in a pre-Cana setting. Rather, it must adapt to the deepening of needs within marriage that arise with time. It goes without saying that the attitude of married couples toward sexuality, children, personal goals and needs, spirituality, and life in general changes dramatically as couples grow in their marriage. How many married couples by their first, tenth, or twenty-fifth anniversary, would say that their view of these issues has not changed from the time they were engaged? The parish must adapt to this change, offering couples dynamic nurturing of their maturing vocation. Pope John Paul II addresses the need for continuous formation of spouses in the lifestyle of NFP as part of the necessary conditions—psychological, moral, spiritual—of living according to God's moral norms:

> But the necessary conditions also include knowledge of the bodily aspect and the body's rhythms of fertility. Accordingly, every effort must be made to render such knowledge accessible to all married people and also to young adults before marriage, through clear, timely and serious instruction and education given by married couples, doctors and experts. Knowledge must then lead to education in self-control: hence the absolute necessity for the virtue of chastity and for *permanent education in it*…

> Married people too are called upon to *progress unceasingly* in their moral life, with the support of a sincere and active desire to gain ever better knowledge of the values enshrined in and fostered by the law of God. They must also be supported by an upright and generous willingness to embody these values in their concrete decisions…On the same lines, it is part of the Church's pedagogy that husbands and wives should first of all recognize clearly the teaching of *Humanae Vitae* as indicating the norm for the exercise of their sexuality, and that they should endeavor to establish conditions necessary for observing that norm (FC 34).

These most important building blocks, marriage and family, are crucial to the life of the parish. Families are the primary source of most of the parish's initiatives and they are certainly the main source of future parishioners and of parish giving. Investing in families is investing in the vitality and future of the parish. Contraception weakens marriages, stunts the growth of families and, in turn, threatens the stability of the parish. Vibrant families make for a vibrant community. It is in the interest of the community to eliminate threats to its welfare.

❼ Pastoral leaders must receive NFP education.

The continuous education of married couples requires an educated leadership:

> This shared progress demands reflection, instruction and suitable education on the part of the priests, religious and lay people engaged in family pastoral work: they will all be able to assist married people in their human and spiritual progress, a progress that demands awareness of sin, a sincere commitment to observe the moral law, and the ministry of reconciliation (FC34).

There are myriad organizations to which pastoral leaders can turn that support NFP education. The starting point should be diocesan NFP coordinators and/or Family Life Coordinators. These offices sometimes organize seminars for priests, create and distribute publications on NFP, and maintain contact information for NFP educators and mission speakers. They can also point inquirers in the direction of organizations that specialize in NFP education such as **One More Soul, Couple to Couple League, Family of the Americas, Billings Ovulation Method Association** and the **Pope Paul VI Institute** to name just a few. CDs and DVDs, pamphlets, magazines, and books are, of course, indispensable in keeping on top of the issue.

The following, although by no means exhaustive, is a standard of resources for self-education:

Audio/Video[40]
- *"Prove it, God"...and He did*, Patty Schneier
- *Why Contraception Matters*, Steve Patton
- *God's Instruction Book on Love and Sex,* Kim Hardy
- *The Spirituality of Responsible Parenthood,* Bishop Salvatore Cordileone

Books[41]
- *Sex and the Marriage Covenant*, John Kippley
- *Love and Responsibility*, Karol Wojtyla (Pope John Paul II)
- *The Art of Natural Family Planning*, by the Couple to Couple League
- *Love and Fertility*, Mercedes Arzu Wilson
- *The Billings Method*, Dr. Evelyn Billings
- *Humanae Vitae: A Generation Later*, Professor Janet E. Smith
- *Good News About Sex and Marriage: Answers to your Honest Questions about Catholic Teaching*, Christopher West
- *Birth Control and Christian Discipleship*, John Kippley

❽ All the little things: literature centers, bulletin announcements, and petitions for General Intercessions.

In order to create an NFP culture in the parish, there must be attention to the little things that, when done consistently, really are not that little. Literature centers placed in the vestibule of the Church, like the checkout isle of a grocery store, give parishioners one last look at what is going on in the parish before they leave to carry Christ out into the world. A little basic marketing can be helpful: pamphlets, flyers, and books must be neat and organized, placed prominently at eye-level, with smart, professional-looking signage and attractive visuals. Effective attention grabbers include, "Is your marriage all it can be?" "What does the Church *really* teach about contraception?", "Marriage builders", "Marriage Insurance", and "Love that Lasts". The *United States Conference of Catholic Bishops* has made posters available in which

---

[40] *One More Soul* offers a tape sampler of 17 tapes that can be assembled a la carte to include the tapes listed here; (800) 307-7685.

[41] All of these titles are available at *One More Soul*. See catalogue for details, or log onto www.OMSoul.com.

[42] USCCB *Diocesan Development Program for NFP*, Tel. 202-541-3240/3070; Fax 202-541-3054; E-mail nfp@usccb.org

the caption, "Capture the Romance," appears underneath a picture of a happy, attractive couple.[42] *One More Soul* distributes ready-made pamphlet packets to get started on a literature center. Personalizing pamphlets with address labels with contact information for local NFP teachers and testimony/consultant couples will direct readers as to where they can dig deeper.

Bulletin announcements are a convenient way to deepen the parish's awareness of NFP. Quotes from notable people in support of NFP, and "factoids" about NFP such as, "Did you know that Natural Family Planning is not the same as the 'Rhythm Method'? Here's why…", or "Did you know that Natural Family Planning has helped infertile couples achieve pregnancy by determining the optimal fertile time for conception?"[43] can get readers thinking. The *U.S. Conference of Catholic Bishops, Diocesan Development Program for NFP* produces a pamphlet called *NFP: Myths and Reality* that debunks misconceptions about NFP with short, pithy snippets; these, also, would be excellent bulletin sections. How about brief personal testimonies from couples who have converted to the NFP lifestyle from a contraceptive lifestyle? *One More Soul* publishes a pamphlet of three such testimonies—entitled "The Hurtful Consequences of Artificial Contraception and Sterilization—that, with regard to both content and length, would be a nice fit for bulletin announcements. A new book from *One More Soul* is also available, entitled *Sterilization Reversal: A Generous Act of Love*, in which twenty Catholic couples share the stories of their reversals. This could be easily adapted for bulletin use by adding whole stories as inserts or by using interesting quotes in the bulletin itself.

The following is a set of notable quotes on NFP/contraception that could be published in bulletins:[44]

- "It was *Humanae Vitae* more than anything else that made me feel I must belong to that Church that could have the extraordinary insight and courage to produce this encyclical—knowing that it would be absolutely torn to pieces, treated as a kind of blasphemy in the idiotic society we live in." *Malcolm Muggeridge*

- "…in some critical respects the abortion decision is of the same character as the decision to use contraception…for two decades people have organized intimate relationships and made choices

---

[43] Second quote, Bernadette Sacksteder.
[44] Compiled by Bernadette Sacksteder.

that define their views of themselves and their place in society, in reliance on the availability of abortion in the event that contraception should fail." *U.S. Supreme Court, Planned Parenthood v. Casey*

- "The close connection which exists, in mentality, between that practice of contraception and that of abortion is becoming increasingly obvious. It is being demonstrated in an alarming way by the development of chemical products, intrauterine devices, and vaccines which, distributed with the same ease as contraceptives, really act as abortifacients in the very early stages of life of a new human being." *Pope John Paul II, Gospel of Life 13*

- "The way to plan the family is Natural Family Planning, not contraception. In destroying the power of giving life, through contraception, a husband or wife is doing something to self. This turns the attention to self, and so it destroys the gift of love in him or her. By properly using the Natural Family Planning method, couples are using their bodies to glorify God in the sanctity of family life." *Mother Teresa*

- "God chooses to bring forth new human life through the love of spouses. God wishes to share His creation with new human souls, and brings new souls into the world through the love of men and women for each other. When a man and woman have a child together, it's an act that changes the cosmos; something has come into existence that will never pass out of existence."*Dr. Janet Smith, Humanae Vitae: A Challenge to Love*

- "NFP allows couples to respect their bodies, obey their God, and fully respect their spouses."
Professor Janet E. Smith, Humanae Vitae: A Challenge to Love

- "The Church condemns contraception not because it wants to deny spouses sexual pleasure, but because it wants to help them find marital happiness and to help them have happy homes, for without these our well-being as individuals and as a society is greatly endangered…In teaching that contraception is intrinsically immoral, the Church is not imposing a disciplinary law on Catholics; she is preaching only what nature and the Gospel preach." *Professor Janet E. Smith, Humanae Vitae: A Challenge to Love*

- "God has entrusted spouses with the extremely important mission of transmitting human life. In fulfilling this mission spouses freely and deliberately render a service to God, the Creator.

> This service has always been a source of great joy, although the joys are, at times, accompanied by not a few difficulties and sufferings." *Humanae Vitae*

- "The experience of tens of thousands of couples has shown that, when lived prayerfully and unselfishly, NFP deepens and enriches marriage and results in great intimacy…and greater joy."
  Archbishop Charles Chaput, Of Human Life

Statistics and study results are eye opening as well. For example, a study sponsored by the Family of the Americas Foundation, a worldwide organization that promotes the ovulation method of NFP, followed 600 NFP-using couples and found that ONLY 0.2 PERCENT OF NFP USERS DIVORCE.[45]

Of course, anything that could be published in the bulletin could be used in the homily. In fact, a tie-in between the homily and bulletin is recommended as a way to draw parishioners' attention to the bulletin item/insert and reinforce their reception of the message from the pulpit.

Some parishes include petitions that accentuate the Church's teaching on the blessings of children and openness to life in the General Intercessions. Indeed the USCCB's *Pastoral Plan for Pro-Life Activities* suggests, "Parishes should include in the petitions at every Mass a prayer that ours will become a nation that respects and protects all human life, born and unborn, reflecting a true culture of life."[46] Saint Boniface parish in Lafayette, Indiana, always includes a petition that contrasts the *culture of death* with the *culture of life*: "That the culture of death, promoting contraception, sterilization, human embryonic research, abortion, infanticide, euthanasia, assisted suicide, capital punishment, and terrorism, would give way to the gospel of life, let us pray to the Lord."

Here are a few more examples:

- For openness among married couples to the gift of life, let us pray to the Lord.

- For all those whose lives have been harmed by abortion, contraception, and sterilization, let us pray to the Lord.

---

[45] Study completed in 2000. Family of the Americas Foundation, 5929 Talbot Rd. Lothian MD 20711
[46] *Pastoral Plan for Pro-Life Activities: A Campaign in Support of Life.* USCCB. Washington, DC: 2001, p. 31.

- For an end to the destructive influence of contraception on marriage, and a renewed openness to the blessings of children, let us pray to the Lord.
- That couples will turn away from reproductive technologies that harm children, such as artificial insemination and in vitro fertilization, let us pray to the Lord.
- That married couples will embrace their fertility and refrain from contraception and sterilization, let us pray to the Lord.
- That the Lord in His mercy would roll back the culture of death and free our land from abortion, contraception, sterilization, and euthanasia, let us pray to the Lord.
- For the young people of our parish and society, that the Lord would protect them from the temptations of contraception and immorality and help them lead full, joyful Christian lives, let us pray to the Lord.
- For all those who have fallen into abortion, contraception, and sterilization, that the Lord would bring them reconciliation and complete healing, let us pray to the Lord.

Priests for Life publishes these petitions:

- *Christmas*: "That the joy of Christmas at the birth of Christ may also be reflected in our willingness to welcome every child, even in difficult circumstances, we pray to the Lord."
- *Feast of the Holy Family*: "That the family may become ever more the sanctuary of life, where all are welcomed as a gift rather than a burden."
- *First Sunday of Lent (A)*: "That all may reject the temptation to 'be like gods' who have mastery over human life, and instead may accept and reverence life as a supreme gift of the Creator, we pray to the Lord."
- *7th Sunday of Easter (A)*: "That as Christ's disciples, who live in a Culture of Death, we may effectively witness the Gospel of Life that has been entrusted to us, we pray to the Lord."
- "That the leaders and members of the Church may fulfill with joy their calling to proclaim, celebrate, and serve the Gospel of Life, we pray to the Lord."

Conclusion

At the 7th annual California Natural Family Planning Conference, March 25, 2000, Father Marcos Gonzalez of St. Andrew Church, Pasadena and Father Roberto Pirrone of Ss. Peter and Paul Church, Wilmington, California, gave testimonies about their experiences with promoting NFP at their parishes. Father Pirrone recounts this story:

> You never know what effect it will have…In my last assignment, Saint Rose of Lima in Maywood, I just mentioned in passing about NFP—*in passing*—and, you know, if we want to go to communion we have to be in a state of grace, and what is mortal sin? It's rejecting God in our lives in various ways, and one of them is the abuse of the gift of marriage. And after Mass this group of people came up to me: "Father, we didn't know that this wasn't in God's will, what are we to do?" This was 35 couples! The modern Catholic is unaware of the Church's teaching. They don't reject it; they don't know it! They've never heard it before and so people are generally open to knowing the truth. They want to have a good marriage.

Father Gonzalez, likewise, has made NFP an integral part of his parish operations. His marriage preparation program requires an Engaged Encounter Retreat, a full, in-house, set of courses in NFP, a multi-course class in the theology of marriage, and a series of one-on-one counseling sessions between himself and prospective spouses. At the time he spoke at the CANFP conference, he had 63 couples in marriage preparation. What a tremendous endorsement for emphasizing NFP in the parish. Far from losing married couples, Father Gonzalez' marriage preparation program is thriving. Father Pirrone explains that there are two moments in which he deals with married couples: in their engagement, when they cannot bear to be apart, and when their marriages are falling apart and they cannot bear to be with each other. "A curious thing," says Pirrone, "when they come in for marriage counseling because of marital problems…I always ask them 'what method of birth control are you using?' 100 percent—now I've only been a priest for six years—but 100 percent of every single couple that I've had with marriage problems is using artificial birth control. I've never had one Natural Family Planning couple, ever, in my office for marriage problems. It just hasn't happened. The divorce rate is the lowest among those who use Natural Family Planning."

Father Randall Moreau, of the diocese of Lafayette, Louisiana, also requires a full set of courses in NFP for prospective couples. He tells the story of how he went from skepticism to enthusiastic advocacy for a full course of NFP for marriage preparation, in a conference that combined his testimony with the testimony of couples who converted to the use of NFP:

> And let me tell you, Fathers, it has worked beautifully. Like you, I had some fears, like, "Is this going to work?" And, "How are people going to react? What are they going to say? Am I just going to lose them all and kind of defeat my purpose here as a priest?"
>
> In my experience, there have been practically no problems, virtually none, and it's really surprised me. Couples have not revolted and refused to go. I never hear "I'm not gonna do that!"
>
> Of course, to be perfectly honest, one of the reasons I have so little problem requiring all four sessions is because my parishioners hear this message from the pulpit and they know ahead of time what the Church teaches on this very crucial issue. I've been here in my current parish for almost four years, and people know where I stand. They've been hearing it from the pulpit consistently. So it's no surprise at all for them to come into my office and expect to hear that they're going to have to go to these Natural Family Planning classes. It's no surprise at all.

Father Moreau reports, moreover, that since he began to enthusiastically promote NFP, parishioners have been more giving of their time, talent and treasure, a phenomenon that he attributes to their greater openness to the will of God. He argues that if a couple is willing to submit this part of their lives to God, there is nothing they will withhold.

Yet this is not an uncommon testimony. Indeed many bishops, priests, and deacons have found that preaching NFP from the pulpit and making instruction in NFP available in the adult education of the diocese and parish has produced overwhelmingly positive results. The office of Natural Family Planning in Saint Cloud, Minnesota, has compiled a cassette tape of testimonials to this fact. Through almost all of these testimonials runs a twofold refrain: (1) that emphasizing NFP and the Church's teaching on contraception builds up the parish, and (2) that feedback from parishioners is almost universally grateful. Father James Sullivan, a Dominican priest asserts, "My overwhelming experience in preaching about contraception [is that it is] readily received. And not only in marriage preparation for engaged couples but also in terms of married couples who struggle with the question of how many children the

Lord is calling them to have...When they hear the truth of the Church's moral teaching, they are naturally drawn to it..."

Catholic Therapist, Deacon Dr. Bob McDonald, likewise reports:

> I've been preaching on contraception from the pulpit for a number of years...At every opportunity I mention contraception. I mention its damaging effects on our relationships as husbands and wives. I mention, of course, the abortifacient probabilities of the contraceptive pill, but also try to make sure that people understand that we're not just talking about the pill but we're talking about a whole variety of techniques which violate [human dignity] and the rights of God in our marriage covenant. That covenant is between husband and wife, yes, but that's not enough. It's between husband, wife, and God. So, indeed, it is a Trinitarian experience, until death do us part.
>
> The result is that my parishioners are appreciative of the preaching that I do. The comment that I hear most frequently is, "Why weren't we told this stuff before? We never heard it! We needed to hear it and we're so glad that you're standing up, being counted, and telling us what the truth is." So have courage...just stand up and do it. Ask the Holy Spirit to guide your words; ask the Holy Spirit to open the hearts of your people. It is the truth that there will be some opposition from one or two individuals, but quite frankly, it is worth it for the Kingdom of God.

The Most Reverend Charles Chaput, Archbishop of Philadelphia, relates similar experience with proclaiming the Church's doctrine on contraception and the blessings of children:

> One of the things I'm constantly surprised about—I would even say astonished—is the number of people who come to talk to me after I've preached about *Humanae Vitae* either directly or as an example within another homily who come and say how grateful they are that I've had the courage to speak about it. My response, almost always, is, "well, it doesn't take any courage because to speak the truth of Christ without compromise is really part of the essential ministry of [a priest and bishop]." So it really shouldn't take extraordinary courage to speak Christ's truth and I've never, in my course of 29 years as a priest, experienced any negative reaction to preaching about *Humanae Vitae* and about the importance of Natural Family Planning for happy married and family life.

While it is absolutely imperative that bishops, priests, and deacons unfold for the faithful the *fullness* of married love, revealing the joy of procreation and the pitfalls of contraception, it is equally necessary that the laity collaborate in this critical ministry. The laity, for whom marriage is the predominant vocation, must witness by word and example to marital chastity and unreserved acceptance of the fruit and pinnacle of married love, children. The truth of the Church's teaching on contraception and procreation is a *gift*, not unlike the Ten Commandments or the Beatitudes, that enables us to live free, fulfilled, and joyful lives. We should no more hesitate to embrace and proclaim this truth than we would hesitate to embrace and proclaim the Golden Rule or love of neighbor. It is part and parcel to living the fullness of the truth in Christ, a universal moral obligation for all who would belong to the Body of Christ. As such, the call of God for us to receive the *totality* of human sexuality belongs to us *all*. The truth about married love and the threat posed to it by contraception cannot, therefore, be relegated to the shadows of private conscience. Nor can it be stowed away as a half-hearted, ten-minute footnote to marriage preparation.

In the final analysis, the issue of contraception and the right ordering of procreation reflects our attitude toward love and life, the virtues on which not only marriage, but the whole of the Gospel, rest. Our world grapples with questions about the transmission of human life that no other generation in history has had to face, forcing us to examine where we stand with regard to love and life. Technology is moving so fast, our world can hardly take time to reflect on its moral implications. Has there ever been a time more suitable for reflection on the meaning of human sexuality and interior examination of our attitude toward God's vision for the transmission of human life? It is time for a renewed catechesis in the proper means and ends of human procreation; time to give these issues—so central not only to the welfare of marriage and family, but to our concept of love and the sanctity of life—prominence in the moral formation of the faithful. Bishop Robert Vasa makes this point particularly well:

> Our modern society has been sold a promise of peaceful, ecstatically happy marital bliss free of responsibility and fear of children, and that promise comes in packages of pills. The Church too promises a life of peaceful, truly joyful marital bliss, but one filled with responsibility and with gratitude for children. One is shallow and sterile; the other is deep, rich, and fertile. Society promises a sterile relationship and that is what people get with society's plan—sterility in relationship. The Church's plan is God's plan, a fruitful plan generating in the hearts of spouses a

rich harvest of generosity and other-centered love. God's plan and grace help to create and foster a life-open relationship wherein spouses see children as gifts of a loving God. Cooperating with God, and not working against Him, is the reason for using Natural Family Planning. A change of heart is needed in our society relative to its view of marital union, children, fidelity, and contraception. I hope this book can play a huge part in helping to bring about that much needed change of heart.[47]

---

[47] Most Reverend Robert F. Vasa, bishop of Santa Rosa, California, letter to the author dated October 30, 2002.

Preaching NFP: Why Not?

By Theresa Notare
Special Assistant of the Diocesan Development Program for NFP (USCCB)

I am often asked "Why don't we hear about Natural Family Planning (NFP) from the pulpit?" The question is practical. Most Catholics agree that husbands and wives need to responsibly plan their families, but few understand why the Church prohibits contraception and few know about NFP. The pulpit may be the best means for Catholics to learn what the Church teaches and why.

Why don't priests preach on NFP? The top three reasons priests give me are:

(1) they must preach on the daily Mass readings;
(2) NFP is an awkward topic for a sermon in a mixed congregation; and
(3) their comfort level may not extend that far.

This third point can take in diverse factors. They may be unfamiliar with the science of NFP. They may have done little serious reading on the theology which supports the use of NFP. They may have no personal friendships with couples who practice NFP, or they may have an innate "shyness" about sexual matters.

I've never met a priest who has rejected the truth of the teachings. I have met some priests who "question" the teachings, but their questions are prompted mostly by a lack of information, not a rejection of the faith.

One priest explained this silence very well: "It's not some conscious clerical plot of silence on the topic," he said. "Priests are practical. They like to speak on issues they know a lot about or have personal experience with. Unless they study, pray, reflect on this issue, and have NFP couples witness to them, they won't get it. They are men; they don't have fertility cycles and aren't married to someone who does. They need help."

What to do? Education. Education. Education. Each of the objections listed above can be overcome by providing clergy with solid information on NFP. The diocesan NFP office is the logical place to start. A diocesan NFP coordinator can plan and implement clergy education. If a diocese does not have an NFP coordinator, interested and informed people can plan activities together and solicit the support of a pastor in a large parish.

Education can take many forms. Direct mailings of brochures or audiotapes can be sent to priests. Full or half-day educational events can be planned. A series of brief lectures can be offered throughout a year. Planned visits to parishes can be scheduled for more candid, one-on-one conversation. Informal dinners should not be overlooked. They can provide a casual atmosphere for significant discussion. Whatever the format, the content of NFP education must address all aspects of the issue: theological/pastoral, scientific/behavioral, and physical/emotional.

First impressions are also critical. Keep in mind that the tone of NFP education should be positive. Say, "God designed human fertility wonderfully so that men and women can join Him in planning their families." Once the good idea has been said, then bring up the negative—"Contraceptive use assaults God's plan for us."

NFP education always must be set within the greater context of the Church's vision of the human person, sexuality, conjugal love and responsible parenthood. When God's design for life and love is presented in all its beauty, it is seen as desirable. When Catholics embrace God's will, they will reject contraception (and other sexually related ills) out of love and understanding.

The science of NFP must be presented with all its strengths and weaknesses, but beginning with NFP's strengths is essential. Few couples understand their combined fertility. NFP provides that education. Research confirms that the Sympto-Thermal and Ovulation methods of NFP are almost 97 percent effective for avoiding pregnancy. Couples need to know this is reliable research.

On the negative side, many couples may find abstinence during the fertile period difficult. NFP teachers need to be sensitive to this. Couples also need to know that NFP "user effectiveness" rates drop to a range from 80 to 90 percent. *This wider range reflects the importance of couple behavior as well as the quality of teaching they received.*

NFP promoters can't do much about a couple's behavior, but improving diocesan NFP services and strengthening the training of NFP teachers is within our reach. All of this can be explained to priests.

Priests also need accurate information on the actions, side effects, and risks of contraceptives. Probably few priests know how these devices and chemicals work and have little understanding of the abortifacient actions of hormonal "contraceptives." Priests need to learn and reflect on how contraceptives negatively affect the physical, emotional and spiritual health of a couple.

Related social issues need to be studied, like the epidemic of sexually transmitted diseases and rates of unintended pregnancies (which often result in abortion). Priests need to see that counseling the individual couple on sexual issues has a public dimension.

When ongoing education on NFP and related issues is offered for priests, the topic will no longer be unpreachable. An informed priest will find many opportunities to preach on NFP in the day's readings. For example, if the readings speak of "God's covenant with the Israelites," he can apply that to the marital covenant whereby a man and a woman become one flesh. It would then be logical to explain why introducing artificial contraception is an affront to that covenant.

If Scripture highlights the problem of worshiping idols, an NFP-educated priest can speak of the false sexual idols which our society promotes. He can preach about the beauty of human sexuality as part of God's plan to give us real freedom and happiness.

When a priest is a friend of an NFP couple, he can share their positive experiences with his congregation. A confident priest knows the ways to provide just enough detail to move his parishioners to listen and to get them to open their hearts.

One last word. Strong NFP educational outreach to priests should include information about where couples can go to learn the methods of NFP. Scheduled classes or home study programs should be made available to all engaged and married couples. NFP education and services go hand in hand.

When all these components work together our priests will be well equipped to help Catholic couples follow God's design for life and love.

Reprinted with permission, Life Issues Forum, a nationally syndicated column, Secretariat for Pro-Life Activities, United States Conference of Catholic Bishops.

A Pastoral Letter on Marriage and the Family

By Most Reverend Harry J. Flynn Archbishop Emeritus of Saint Paul and Minneapolis

Following the command and example of Jesus Christ, the Catholic Church proclaims that "by (God's) plan man and woman are united, and married life is established as the one blessing not forfeited by original sin nor washed away in the flood" (Nuptial Blessing from Marriage Ceremony). The very life of God is manifested in marriage, for He "has made the union of man and woman so holy a mystery that it symbolizes the marriage of Christ and His Church." In such powerful language the Church thus announces God's intention that marriage play a crucial role in His plan for human happiness. It has been the strong and constant teaching of the Catholic Church that the family is the foundation of all human society and the irreplaceable institution for the education and formation of children.

Even as we rejoice in the beauty and dignity of marriage, however, we must also acknowledge that we live in a society in which marriage is misunderstood and even denigrated. Vows have been frequently broken. The gift of life has been rejected. Cohabitation before marriage has clouded the intrinsic connection between marriage vows and physical sexual union, thus undermining the character of marital fidelity and the virtue of chastity. Divorce has caused great damage to human relationships and especially to the emotional and spiritual health of children, as they so frequently experience the painful absence of a parent from their lives.

The purpose of this pastoral letter is not specifically to discuss such problems and difficulties, although the Church understands the urgent needs which result from them and, thankfully, already has a number of programs which address them. Rather, in this letter, I wish to focus on those means by which our Church can provide a truly useful and Catholic program of preparation for marriage. Such programs need to prepare men and women for their God-given vocation by helping them recognize their call to holiness, understand the dignity of the sacrament they will receive, and make the necessary commitment that will allow their marriage to be faithful and fruitful.

From the beginning, God intended the union of husband and wife—characterized by mutual fidelity, lifelong commitment, and openness to the transmission of life—to be the sign on earth of His love of His people.

This nuptial symbolism pervades Sacred Scripture. The marriage of man and woman reflects the very nature of the Trinitarian God by Whose love the world was created and is sustained. Fulfilling the demands of Christian marriage in joyful fidelity gives witness to the essential goodness of God's creation and invites participation in the creative plan of God. Marriage and family life are not only the foundation of human society but also one of the surest means of preaching the Gospel and evangelizing the world. Thus, husbands, wives, and their children share more fully in this mystery of salvation.

The preparation for a fruitful sacramental marriage begins early in life. Children daily experience the relationship between their parents; the love, care, and consideration that husbands and wives display for each other; and the way in which they welcome and nurture children. These experiences leave a lasting impression on the consciousness of those children and affect their attitudes toward marriage and family life. Gradually, as the children mature, they are provided with a careful catechesis regarding the nature of marriage, the mystery of human sexuality, the inherent value of human life, and the practice of virtue. The manner in which both Jesus and St. Paul speak about marriage and celibacy in tandem suggest that the virtue of chastity is the context in which both states of life are best understood, for it is in purity of heart that we shall see God. This general, family-oriented preparation will flourish in an atmosphere of fidelity to the life of Christ and His commands, in which prayer and spiritual sacrifice are central.

In addition to the general preparation for marriage and family life just described, a couple also needs to participate in an intense, very personal preparation during the 12 months immediately prior to the actual celebration of the sacrament. Therefore, we turn now to a consideration of certain elements which form the core of an authentic preparation for Catholic marriage. Many existing programs for marriage preparation instruct couples in the realities of financial planning, interpersonal communication, career expectations, and other sociological aspects of marriage. To enable them to accomplish this work in the most effective fashion, these programs enlist the help of experienced married couples who generously offer their time and wisdom to encourage younger men and women preparing to marry. Such elements undoubtedly make a valuable contribution to a couple's preparation for marriage and should continue to be included. It is of far greater importance, however, that preparation place particular emphasis on the specifically religious and sacramental elements involved in the beautiful vocation of marriage.

If couples understand the nature of a vow, in both its religious and personal meaning, and grasp the nature of the sacraments rooted in the sacrificial death and resurrection of Jesus Christ, they will more readily approach marriage as a lifelong commitment to the service of spouse, children, and family. This is a commitment that entails no small measure of sacrifice even as it brings fulfillment.

Each couple should clearly realize the fundamental unity of marriage and family life and be prepared to welcome children as the supreme gift of marriage. In marriage, a couple is "ordained" to the teaching and moral formation of children. Within the "domestic Church" of the family, the husband and wife awaken their children to the reality of their human dignity and eternal destiny. How important, then, it is that the couple preparing for marriage possess a firm knowledge of their faith and bear witness to their intent to practice that faith in their marriage and family life. This preparation will flourish in an atmosphere nurtured by the weekly celebration of the death and resurrection of Jesus Christ in the Eucharist, and by the frequent reception of the sacrament of Penance, through which persons learn that forgiveness which is so vital to human relationships.

A marriage program would not be complete if it did not promote the proper understanding of the human person, made in the image of God, and called to eternal life. It is important that couples seeking to marry understand that they fulfill their vocation in bodily as well as spiritual ways. The practice of virtues, particularly chastity, forms a necessary prerequisite to an enduring and faithful marriage. A firm grasp of the Church's teaching on human sexuality is essential, as is the understanding that marriage is the preeminent way by which their baptismal vocation to holiness is lived out. Every marriage program also ought to introduce couples to Natural Family Planning. Natural Family Planning honors the Catholic teaching on the indissoluble link between life and love, provides a way by which husbands and wives come to understand each other more intimately, and offers an escape from the contraceptive mentality that threatens to corrupt marriages and all interpersonal relationships.

Though it does not properly fall under the heading of marriage preparation, I also wish to note briefly the great need for post wedding help for young couples, especially within the first years of marriage. Such topics as the movement from personal to familial spirituality, the art of communication, the development of a healthy and chaste sexual expression, the preparation for the arrival of children, and a variety of practical adjustments as the "two become one" are all of concern. Newly married couples are challenged to live a deeply spiritual commitment in the midst of a social and political atmosphere in which human life is threatened by abortion, violence, and a general disregard for the inherent value of the human person. Particularly as they begin their new life together, these couples need our support, our encouragement, and our assistance.

As I conclude this reflection, I also want to offer a word of encouragement to those Catholics who are living in a difficult marriage or are enduring the distress of a broken marital relationship. Our Lord was no stranger to suffering, nor was He distant from those in confusion and pain. I want to assure anyone with marital difficulties of the Church's continued desire to offer you the solace of Christ, to work with you to resolve your difficulties, and ease your distress. There are a number of programs available to assist those in troubled marriages or those who are separated and divorced. They should never feel separated from the community of the Church, even though the emotional burden that they carry may be heavy.

In this pastoral letter, I have shared with you some key ideas intended to assist men and women entering into marriage to do so with knowledge, commitment, maturity, confidence, and joy. In such marriages, husbands and wives will answer their call to holiness and fulfill their baptismal vocation to transform the world according to the pattern of Christ. In such marriages, a culture of life will prevail, in which children are welcomed generously and given an environment in which they can grow in the knowledge and love of God. Through such marriages, we will all be blessed, since they will provide a clear and shining sign of the love and fidelity of Jesus Christ for His people.

Pastoral Recommendations

In order to help ensure that all those preparing for marriage understand the great dignity of their vocation, I am calling upon all parish-based and Archdiocesan marriage courses to address the following elements:

I. A clear understanding and vision of the sacramental nature of Christian marriage, including, but not limited to:

- A Christian understanding of the human person
- A redemption of man and woman in Christ
- How marriage is a reflection of Christ's love for the Church
- A practical understanding of the Canonical promises–fidelity, permanence,
  openness to life.

II. A clear understanding of the Church's teaching on human sexuality, including:

- Instruction on NFP–at least two introductory classes
- Understanding of the morality of various reproductive technologies

III. Marriage preparation will begin at least one year and not less than six months prior to the wedding date. A minimum of five sessions with a priest, deacon or other qualified person or couple. This should include a Marriage Inventory and subsequent discussions of the results.

IV. Encourage parishes and current marriage preparation providers to develop ongoing programs and support for newly married couples especially in the first three years. This may include a series of classes or parish day of reflection.

Finally, all of these pastoral recommendations will only be fruitful to the extent that a couple develops their own relationship with the person of Christ through prayer, forgiveness, and service.

Most Reverend Harry J. Flynn
Archbishop of Saint Paul and Minneapolis

Appendix
Homily Guide
Homilies

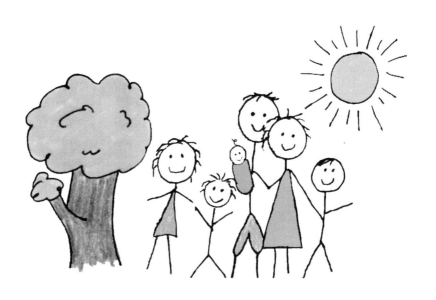

The Pill, the Pope, the Problem p. 141

Fr. Walter Austin, Our Lady of the Lake Parish, Mandaville, Louisiana

15th Sunday, Ordinary Time, Cycle A ▶ Is 55:10-11; Rom 8:18-23; Mt 13:1-23.

Summary: Father Austin comments on the authoritative quality of Humanae Vitae, its historical context, and its wisdom. He addresses the negative social impact of contraception and briefly outlines the function and benefits of Natural Family Planning. Included in his explanation of NFP is the difference between contraception and NFP.

Proclaiming Truth in and out of Season p. 145

Fr. John Bateman, Saint Joseph Catholic Church, Hanover, Pennsylvania

20th Sunday, Ordinary Time, Cycle C ▶ Jer 38:4-6, 8-10; Heb 12:1-4; Lk 12:49-53.

Summary: The Church, like Jeremiah and Jesus, is unwilling to compromise the truth to bring about a counterfeit peace. Her teaching on contraception is no exception; she continues to be a source of division and conflict because she proclaims the truth of married love in its wholeness, despite widespread rejection of this truth.

"Woman, How Great Is Your Faith!" p. 150

Fr. Phillip Bloom, Holy Family Parish, Seattle, Washington

20th Sunday, Ordinary Time, Cycle A ▶ Is 56:1, 6-7; Rom 11:13-15, 29-32; Mt 15:21-28.

Summary: Contraception depersonalizes those who use it, in much the same way that the Canaanites and the other Gentiles had been depersonalized during Jesus' time. In keeping with Jesus' example of promoting the human dignity of individuals, we must promote means of family planning that preserve this dignity. The Church seeks to heal those hurt by contraception and stands against approaches to family planning that exploit women.

Seek and You Shall Find: The Beauty of Humanae Vitae   p. 153

Fr. McLean Cummings, Diocese of Baltimore, On Assignment with Aid to Russia

17th Sunday, Ordinary Time, Cycle C ▶ Gn 18:20-32; Col 2:12-14; Lk 11:1-13.

Summary: On the 30th anniversary of Humanae Vitae, Father Cummings considers some of the negative social effects of contraception—promiscuity, divorce, and abortion—while highlighting the positive impact of NFP on marriage and family life.

Children Make Us More Human   p. 156

Fr. Brian Doerr, Director of Vocations, Diocese of Lafayette, Indiana

13th Sunday, Ordinary Time, Cycle A ▶ 2 Kgs 4:8-11, 14-16; Rom 6:3-4, 8-11; Mt 10:37-42.

·Summary: Selfishness and consumerism have cast children as rivals to a carefree, hedonistic lifestyle. Children crush our selfishness, teaching us to grow in self-sacrificial love.

Revisiting Humanae Vitae   p. 160

Most Reverend John F. Donoghue, DD, Archbishop of Atlanta

16th Sunday, Ordinary Time, Cycle C ▶ Gn 18:1-10; Col 1:24-28; Lk 10:38-42.

Summary: Archbishop Donoghue addresses the negative consequences of "man's arrogant assumption of the management of life, which began with [contraception]." The homily concludes on a hopeful note, that is, Mary and Martha show us that the culture can be transformed by receiving Christ.

God's Plan for Human Life   p. 164

Fr. Matthew Habiger, OSB, PhD, St. Benedict's Abbey, Atchison, Kansas

7th Sunday of Easter, Cycle C ▶ Acts 7:55-60; Rv 22:12-14, 16-17, 20; Jn 17:20-26.

Summary: Fr. Habiger reflects on the Easter mystery as a lesson in God's plan for life. The Incarnation reveals to us the importance of our bodies as signs of our interior life. Christ showed us his divine, life-giving love bodily by dying and rising. In contrast, contraception signifies bodily what the heart does not mean, thereby falsifying the inner truth of married love. Easter grace gives us hope for repenting of unchastity and pleasing God by living lives of authentic love.

Trinity Sunday Homily   p. 168

Fr. Matthew Habiger, OSB, PhD, St. Benedict's Abbey, Atchison, Kansas

Trinity Sunday, Cycle A ▶ Ex 34:4-6, 8-9; 2 Cor 13:11-13; Jn 3:16-18.

Summary: Marriage, as a communion of persons, is a sign of the Trinity. Just as the persons of the Trinity share self-emptying love, so, too, must spouses offer themselves fully to one another. Contraception is an obstacle to this complete mutual self-gift.

The Church's Moral Teaching on Contraception (a series of 3 sermons)

Fr. Anthony Kopp, O Praem, St. Michael's Abbey, Norbertine Fathers of Orange County

(1) 23rd Sunday, Ordinary Time, Cycle A ▶ Ez 33:7-9; Rom 13:8-10; Mt 18:15-20   p. 171

Summary: Fr. Kopp considers the Biblical foundations of the Church's teaching on contraception and emphasizes the importance of trusting the teaching authority of the Church as it is animated by the Holy Spirit.

(2) 25th Sunday, Ordinary Time, Cycle A ▶ Is 55:6-9; Phil 1:20-24, 27; Mt 20:1-16   p. 176

Summary: In keeping with the theme of the readings for this Sunday—God's generosity—Father Kopp teaches that parents must be generous in their family planning. Using Vatican II's Gaudium et Spes (Pastoral Constitution on the Church in the Modern World), he answers a question raised in part 1 of his three-part series: "How many children should a married couple have?"

(3) Respect Life Sunday, 27th Sunday, Ordinary Time, Cycle A ▶ Is 5:1-7; Phil 4:6-9; Mt 21:33-43.   p. 180

Summary: Implicit in this homily are the themes of the day's readings: Paul's emphasis on purity of thought (chastity), and the need for repentance in the face of God's judgment in the parable of the tenant farmers. Reflecting on paragraph 2370 of the Catechism of the Catholic Church, Father Kopp answers a question raised in part 2 of his series: "If it is licit, for grave reasons, to postpone pregnancy, what means must we use?" Father explains the benefits of NFP and explains the difference between NFP and contraception.

Anti-life Message Finds a Home in Contraception
p. 186

Most Reverend Paul S. Loverde, DD, STL, JCL Bishop of Arlington, Virginia

Solemnity of the Birth of John the Baptist ▶ Is 49:1-6; Acts 13:22-26; Lk 1:57-66, 80.

Summary: Bishop Loverde explains the close connection contraception has to abortion and highlights three ways to preserve the morality of the marital act, the cause for which John the Baptist was martyred.

Love Means Giving Oneself Away
p. 189

Most Reverend Thomas J. Olmsted, Bishop of Wichita, Kansas

Anniversary of Roe v. Wade, 2nd Sunday, Ordinary Time, Cycle A ▶ Is 49:3, 5-6; 1 Cor 1:1-3; Jn 1:29-34.

Summary: In a homily given on the weekend before the anniversary of Roe v. Wade, Bishop Olmsted discusses the difference between authentic and counterfeit love. Love as self-gift is exemplified in Christ's "This is my body given up for you," whereas the contraceptive mentality and its ultimate end, abortion, use the phrase, "This is my body," in a self-serving way. There is reason for hope, however, in that while all counterfeits will pass away, genuine love will always remain.

Mass Commemorating the 30th Anniversary of Humanae Vitae p. 193

Justin Cardinal Rigali, JCD, Archbishop emeritus of Philadelphia

13th Sunday, Ordinary Time, Cycle C ▶ 1 Kgs 19:16, 19-21; Gal 5:1, 13-18, Lk 9:51-62.

Summary: Cardinal Rigali outlines the harmful effects of contraception on the modern world. He holds that "joyfully and faithfully living the vision of Christian marriage and family" is the antidote to the contraceptive culture.

Perceiving the Contraception Connection p. 198

Fr. Raymond Suriani, St. Pius X Church, Westerly, Rhode Island

2nd Sunday, Ordinary Time, Cycle A ▶ Is 49:3, 5-6; 1 Cor 1:1-13 Jn 1:29-34.

Summary: Like John the Baptist, we are called to see beneath the surface of things—to look deeper. We are expected to see the false promises of contraception—its harms and its connection to the culture of death, especially the evil of abortion.

"This Sort of Talk Is Hard to Endure! How Can Anyone Take It Seriously?" p. 202

Fr. Joseph Taphorn, Archdiocese of Omaha, Nebraska

21st Sunday, Ordinary Time, Cycle B ▶ Jos 24:1-2, 15-17, 18; Eph 5:21-32; Jn 6:60-69.

Summary: Like the Apostles, who remained with Jesus after the Bread of Life discourse while the rest of his disciples departed, we are asked to embrace the Church's teaching on contraception and marital love even though many around us have rejected it.

The Pill, the Pope, the Problem

By Father Walter Austin
Our Lady of the Lake Parish, Mandaville, Louisiana

"When the disciples got near him, they asked him, 'Why do you speak in parables?' He answered: 'To you has been given the knowledge of the mysteries of the reign of God, but it has not been given to the others. To the man who has, more will be given until he grows rich; the man who has not, will lose what little he has. I use parables when I speak to them because they look but do not see, they listen but do not hear or understand.'" (Matt. 13:10-13)

Jesus uses parables to teach. Though the parables of Jesus date back two thousand years we find a timelessness about them. As we grow in maturity of faith, we get more insight from them.

We can say the same about the teachings of the Church. For nearly two thousand years, the Church has given to the community of believers a body of teachings that helps explain and guide us in living the ways of faith. At times, some of us may find difficulty in comprehending why the Church teaches as it does. However as we look back we can see the wisdom of that teaching and why we believe the Holy Spirit guides the Magisterium or teaching authority of the Church.

In July 1968, Pope Paul VI issued the encyclical *Humanae Vitae* (concerning Human Life). Recall that pivotal year of 1968. In our country the war in Vietnam raged on with no end in sight. Students on our college campuses protested the war and challenged all authority. Our cities burned from racial violence. We witnessed the assassination of men like Dr. Martin Luther King and Robert Kennedy. Riots broke out at the Democratic Convention in Chicago. Lax moral conduct became the sexual revolution. The watchword among youth fascinated by the effects of hallucinatory drugs was, "Tune in, turn on, drop out."

The world witnessed war and revolution. The Soviets invaded Czechoslovakia ending a brief stint with democracy. The cold war raged on as the threat of nuclear annihilation affected our lives. The Church following Vatican II struggled with an explosion of radical changes and ideas. Historians consider 1968 a pivotal year in 20th century history. In this year of turbulence Pope Paul VI issued his papal encyclical on the regulation of human birth: *Humanae Vitae*. "THE POPE BANS THE PILL" ran the newspaper headlines. Catholics who preferred to get their information from a biased secular press overreacted. In Washington, D.C. some Catholics walked out of Mass at the cathedral as the archbishop tried to explain this complex document. Many Catholics had made up their minds and would not listen to the pope or the teaching of the Church. Now a generation later we can look back and evaluate the wisdom of this teaching.

The document begins with the statement "the most serious duty of transmitting human life, for which married persons are the free and responsible collaborators of God the Creator, has always been a source of great joy to them even if sometimes accompanied by not a few difficulties and by distress."

God is the creator of all life. Married couples collaborate with God by bringing human life into the world. They provide a long term stable environment for the development and nurturing of that life. Raising a family is not easy but at the same time children provide tremendous joy to couples who open themselves to life.

Married couples express their mutual love especially in the marital act, which opens itself to the possibility of new life. These two elements of conjugal love and life are two inseparable aspects of marriage. The problem with the artificial use of birth control is that it separates the sex act from the openness to life. Proponents of artificial birth control argued in 1968 that married couples would experience happier and more stable marriages once they were free of the tension over an unwanted pregnancy. They argued that this would result in fewer divorces. However, in the past generation our divorce rate has escalated to over 50% of all marriages. These same advocates added that artificial birth control would result in fewer out-of-wedlock pregnancies. Today the single-parent mother has become the new poverty class in the U.S. We have millions of babies born out of wedlock despite the easy availability of artificial birth control.

Humanae Vitae did not condone couples in marriage having children without responsibility. Couples could space children: "If, then, there are serious motives to space out births, which derive from the physical or psychological conditions of husband and wife, or from external conditions, the Church teaches that it is then licit to take into account the natural rhythms immanent in the generative functions, for the use of marriage in the infecund periods only, and in this way to regulate birth without offending [these] moral principles."

This method of family planning which employs the natural periods of infertility in the woman's ovulation cycle, often draws snickers from

Catholics who recall the old rhythm method. For many couples this method did not work. New methods such as the Sympto-Thermal Method provide couples with a safe means of expressing their love in the marriage act while avoiding an unplanned pregnancy. This natural method differs radically from artificial birth control in its effects and intent.

In NFP the couple chooses to abstain from the marital act when it would not be prudent for them to conceive another child. They do nothing to prevent a new human life from beginning in a freely chosen marital act. They choose to engage in the marital act when the wife is not fertile because this act has purposes other than procreation.

Contracepting couples, on the other hand, choose to engage in sexual union, reasonably anticipating that by doing so new human life will begin. They choose to do something, prior to, during, or subsequent to this freely chosen marital act precisely to prevent this life from beginning. They do not open themselves to the possibilities of new life and remove God from the process.

While the document stresses the cause and effect of the evils of artificial birth control, I find the most prophetic words in the document are, "it is also to be feared that the man, growing used to the employment of anti-conception practices, may finally lose respect for the woman and, no longer caring for her physical and psychological equilibrium, may come to the point of considering her as a mere instrument of selfish enjoyment, and no longer as his respected and beloved companion."

I have seen confirmation of these words in my work with high school girls. Girls feel pressured into premarital sex by both boyfriends and female peers. I recall a junior in high school asking me in front of her class, "Is it a sin to have sex with your boyfriend if you don't enjoy it?" I told her to think about what she asked me. If her boyfriend pressures her into unwanted sex then maybe she should drop him as a boyfriend. If her friends pressured her to prove herself as a woman by engaging in unwanted sex then maybe they are not very good friends.

Women as sex objects rather than as partners in a love relationship goes beyond the high school years. I see it in the ever-increasing tendency for couples to enter into non-committal live-in relationships. Why get married and have children if the sexual aspect of married life can be fulfilled while avoiding any of the responsibilities? We live in a society that avoids long-term commitments. Why commit yourself to someone who will readily meet your needs without such a commitment?

As Catholics the Church asks us to trust its teachings. *Humanae Vitae* is no exception. Look at the results of the past few decades. We find that over 50% of all marriages in the U.S. end in divorce. Yet in 92% of those divorced marriages we find that either one or both of the parties do not practice their religion. That divorce rate reflects the numbers of Catholics divorcing as well. Studies show that married couples who have a strong religious faith produce marriages with the greatest degree of fulfillment.

Recent history reflects the fact that many of the warnings the pope mentions in *Humanae Vitae* have come true. Women have lost their special place as partners in a loving marital relationship and as collaborators in procreation and have found themselves in the unenviable position of sex objects.

Proponents of artificial birth control argued in 1968 that with the fear of pregnancy diminished, women could engage in sex freely without consequences. A generation later we find divorces at an all time high, sexually transmitted diseases ravaging our nation and the effects of broken marriages affecting our youth.

When the Church teaches, we must assume that it teaches what God expects of us. When we choose to go our own way we unfortunately must pay the price for our sins. Those who pay the price are not just those who willingly disregard such teaching but the innocent as well.

Jesus gave to the apostles and the Church the *"mysteries of the reign of God."* As the Church shares with us these mysteries we recall the words of Jesus: *"But blest are your eyes because they see and blest are your ears because they hear"* (Matt. 13:16). Over the past few decades, many Catholics in their blindness and deafness have chosen to ignore this teaching of the Church. We can only wonder what our society might be like today if people had listened to that teaching in 1968.

Proclaiming Truth in and out of Season

By Father John Bateman
Saint Joseph Catholic Church, Hanover, Pennsylvania

You all just did an amazing thing, and you probably don't even realize you did it. I just proclaimed a Gospel that says, "Jesus said to his apostles, I come not for peace, but for division. Mother shall be against daughter and father against son." And when I finished the Gospel I announced it by saying "The Gospel of the Lord." And you all responded, "Praise to you, Lord Jesus Christ." Praise to you for *this* reading? Are you crazy?! Thank you, Jesus, for giving us words of division and strife and difficulty! Really? Yes! You proclaimed, "Praise to you Lord, and thank you for giving us these words, for proclaiming yourself an object of division, not of peace." But what kind of peace is Jesus talking about? What division does He refer to? Well, it's not the peace that this world knows. We need to understand what kind of peace and division Jesus speaks about today. Our readings wonderfully explain to us exactly what division and peace Jesus is talking about, and it begins in today's first reading.

The prophet Jeremiah…To understand this reading, we must first put it into context. Jeremiah was one called by God to proclaim and speak God's word to His people, Israel. He was called by God while he was still very young. In his early days, Jeremiah, faithful to God's word, proclaimed peace and prosperity and joy to the people of Israel. He was loved by the people and by the king because he spoke words of great comfort and hope to the people. But, as time passed, a new king came to power who was not as faithful to God as was the previous one. At the same time, Israel was invaded by Assyria, so they were living as a people in occupation. The faith of the Hebrews did not agree with that of the Assyrians, and they began to suffer greatly under their oppressors. In order to bring about peace in the land, the king of Israel began to make some concessions to his occupying force. "OK, we'll give in on this point of faith, if you will stop sending invading armies into our territory. We'll give in on this matter of faith if you will just give us food when we are hungry." In order to bring about peace and stability, the king of Israel gave in on important matters of faith and began to water it down.

Jeremiah witnessed all this and, still faithful to God's word, proclaimed to the king and to all the people of Israel what the Lord God said. Rather than words of comfort and prosperity, Jeremiah spoke words of doom. "O

King, you and the entire nation of Israel will suffer greatly and be destroyed for your lack of faith and trust in the Lord God." The king and the people no longer liked what Jeremiah had to say. He was despised because he no longer spoke comforting words, but words of destruction. He was hated by the people because they didn't like what they heard.

So, as we hear in today's reading, they lowered Jeremiah into the cistern so that he might die. They told Jeremiah to stop speaking words of ill, because he was demoralizing the troops who were there to protect them. He refused to be silent because he was speaking God's word. For this, they put him in the cistern to die—because he proclaimed the truth of God's words—and the people didn't like it. Jeremiah, at the beginning of his ministry as prophet, spoke words of truth that the people liked, but once that word became more difficult, they hated him, even though he still spoke God's word. He became a source, not of peace, but of division among the people. This is what Jesus is talking about.

Jesus Himself was a source of division and conflict. The Jewish leaders did not want to hear what Jesus had to say. Yet, He persisted in speaking the truth. He could, at any moment, have decided that the risks were too great, the ridicule too excessive. He could have decided to speak other words, words that were not true, and so save His life. But He knew that He must remain faithful to God's word, despite disfavor, opposition, and possible death. We must do the same.

The Church today continues to be a source of conflict and division among the peoples of the world. It is always interesting to watch reactions when the Pope or the Church makes a statement on morality. Many in the world begin to laugh and ridicule the Church, saying things like, "Oh my, those bunch of old men in Rome don't have any idea what reality is. They should just get with the times and leave the Middle Ages—after all, it's the 21st century! Don't they know that?" The Church, in her pronouncements, becomes a source of conflict and division, not only in the secular world, but also for many within the Church. And yet, she continues to speak what she knows to be the truth. She never concedes to the pressures and influences of society to water down the truth or back away from it because it is too difficult. The Church consistently proclaims the truth.

There are many examples of this. Here's one. *Humanae Vitae* was an encyclical published some 30 years ago. In it, after consultation with special commissions, his own theologians and the People of God, Pope Paul VI proclaimed (infallibly) that artificial birth control is intrinsically evil and not permissible. Many immediately scoffed and ridiculed the Church and Paul VI for his outdated thinking. However, we have come, in the course of these 30 odd years, to see the truth of what Paul proclaimed. The proponents and supporters of contraceptives had made certain claims. But Paul VI prophetically spoke of them saying effectively, "If you accept as your truth that artificial contraceptives are okay, there are some grave consequences to that error."

For example, the supporters of contraception boldly proclaimed that allowing their use would reduce the number of unwanted pregnancies. Paul VI said no. He has proven to be correct. In a 1996 article in *U.S. News and World Report,* it was reported that in 1995 there were 1.4 million abortions in this country and 4 million births. Some 25 years after contraceptives were accepted by many in society, the number of unwanted children has *not* been reduced. When 25% of those conceived are murdered through abortion, have we truly reduced the number of unwanted pregnancies? No, we've just killed them. Paul VI stated that if contraceptives were permitted, women would suffer great harm to their very dignity as persons. The supporters of birth control, on the other hand, predicted that contraceptives would finally give women control and "reproductive rights" equal with that of men. Has this happened? No. Women are now treated with far less respect than they were. Men can now look at women, not as human persons with dignity and honor that should be cherished, but rather as objects of their desires. Women have become mere objects, and not the fully emancipated persons so many predicted. Many women bought this false prediction hook, line and sinker, and now they allow themselves to be treated, not with dignity and respect, but as mere objects—to be used and then thrown away.

I believe that after three decades, we can look back to Paul VI and say, "*Humanae Vitae* was right! Paul VI was right!" Despite all the negative publicity the Church took for this encyclical and teaching, she nevertheless continued, and still continues, to proclaim the truth that artificial birth control is intrinsically evil. Many in the secular world, and even in the Church, could not accept this. Even prominent Catholic theologians publicly denounced the Church's teaching. But the past several decades have proven that Paul VI was right. The Church, despite all that she suffered, continued to teach the truth.

There are many other examples, just within *Humanae Vitae*, but there are other teachings of the Church which are just as unpopular in society today, and for which the Church is ridiculed and is a source of division and conflict in our world. For example, the current debate on stem-cell research. President Bush, while he was in Rome, went to see the Holy Father and asked his opinion. I can imagine that Pope John Paul II said to him, "Dubya, no! It is morally wrong!" "But how can this be so?", many ask, "There can be such great medical advances as a result of this research." True, there could be, but we must focus on a much more basic concept—the dignity of every human person from the moment of conception. At conception, there is a separate vulnerable and dependant life, which differs from both mother and father. There is a new life, which is present in every embryo. To do research on embryonic stem cells, we must kill and destroy this new life. We must violate every core principle of the dignity of human life. This cannot be allowed. It's a very dangerous area. So, are we not to have scientific progress? Of course we are, but with restraint and respect for life. The question becomes so arbitrary. I have a bad heart; shall we kill our lector who has a good heart in order that I could have it? What about one of our Special Ministers of Holy Communion, how about one of our servers—couldn't I get one of their hearts? The question, who lives and who dies in the name of scientific research or progress or treatment of ills becomes very arbitrary, and very dangerous.

Many other teachings of the Church continue to be a source of conflict and division in the world and in the Church. The teachings on homosexuality, pre-marital sex, cohabitation, capital punishment, euthanasia, the Church's documents on economic justice or the rights of third world countries and indebtedness are all teachings that are ridiculed, at best, if not completely ignored, because the world doesn't like what it hears. Too bad! It's the truth, and the Church will continue to proclaim it, in season and out of season. The Church, I have come to firmly believe, proclaims the truth to us—a truth that, at times, is very difficult to understand and perhaps very difficult to live out—but it is truth nonetheless. These are truths which *must* be proclaimed. The Church, like Jeremiah, like Jesus Himself, is unwilling to compromise the truth to bring about peace. She continues to be a source of division and of conflict because she proclaims the truth that has been revealed to us.

Let's face it, some Church teachings are extremely difficult. They even cause great conflict and division within us. "How can this be so?" we ask ourselves. Yet the Church persists in proclaiming the truth. I'll be honest, while I was in seminary, I chose to do a concentration in morality, not so that I could boldly proclaim what the Church taught, but so that I, along with the rest of the world, could say, "Oh, come on! We're living in the modern world now not the 1200's!" But, through study and prayer and being open to the Spirit, I have come to believe firmly that what the Church teaches *is* indeed the truth and we cannot compromise it, or we risk loosing everything, even eternal life. Many of us struggle with issues, with various teachings of the Church, and that's okay, so long as we are striving to understand why the Church teaches as she does. It may take an entire lifetime just to begin to understand something the Church teaches; that's okay. But we must, in all things, seek the truth and strive to live it.

To be in error about the truth is one thing. To know the truth and do or proclaim otherwise is another. We know the truth. The Church proudly and pastorally proclaims the truth—we have it! But do we choose to ignore it? Beware. We are falling into the trap. Like Jesus, like Jeremiah, we must boldly proclaim the truth without fear of what others will say or what will happen to us. We must be signs of contradiction, sources of division and conflict in our world by the way that we proclaim and live the truth in our lives.

Okay, this is extremely serious and difficult stuff, but Jesus, in the beginning of today's Gospel, gives us words of great hope and encouragement. "I have come to bring fire to the earth, and how I wish it was ablaze!" What's He talking about? What fire? Don't you remember the day of Pentecost, when those 12 scared and frightened men gathered in the upper room were filled with the Holy Spirit? "And tongues as of fire appeared over each of their heads and they were filled with the Holy Spirit." Suddenly these men who were fearful for their very lives were out in the streets boldly proclaiming Christ crucified. We were filled with that same Spirit on the day of our baptism and given the same mission of being signs of contradiction, sources of conflict in our world by proclaiming the truth. In the sacrament of confirmation, we were filled with those Gifts of the Spirit (wisdom, knowledge, courage, fear of the Lord) so that *we* could go out, boldly, and proclaim the truths of Jesus.

Jesus did not come to bring about a peace that is concession and that forgoes truth to get along. Jesus came to bring us the Truth, and it is our mission, as baptized members of Christ's Body, to proclaim and live that truth in our lives. Perhaps as we come forward today, as we come to this altar of sacrifice to be nourished and strengthened by Christ's Body and Blood, we need to pray along with Jesus that the fire of the Holy Spirit would be enkindled in us, and in all the world. We must pray that we will have the courage to boldly speak the truth, not to water it down, not to make concessions, but to live and proclaim the truth in our own lives. May the fire of the Spirit be enkindled in each of us, that we, like Jeremiah, like Jesus, boldly proclaim the truth, no matter what the cost, no matter what the conflict. If we do this, then the world will truly know peace—not the world's peace, but the peace which only God can give, the peace of His truth.

"Woman, How Great Is Your Faith!"

By Father Phil Bloom
Holy Family Parish, Seattle, Washington

Father Phil Bloom served as a Maryknoll priest associate in Peru from 1987 to 1994. He has founded a Family Planning Center named for his mother, Mary Bloom. The Mary Bloom Center, which includes a small clinic, continues to teach married couples and health professionals in the Billings Method of Natural Family Planning.

Today we hear about one of the truly magnificent women of the Gospel. She was a Canaanite (a pagan people surrounding Israel) and she had one goal: the healing of her daughter who was gripped by a demon. When Jesus passed through her territory, she pled her case with him. The disciples wanted to stop her, even Jesus seemed to brush her aside: "It is not right to take the food of the children and give it to the dogs."

Here is where we see her true greatness. She could have been discouraged, she could have been sidetracked by a seeming offense and said: "Don't call me a dog." But the word "dog" admits a positive as well as negative sense, like in English we speak for example about a "lucky dog." So she took it in the best sense and said, "Yes, Lord, but even the dogs eat the crumbs which fall from their master's table."

And she received from Jesus his highest praise: "Woman, your faith is great!" And he healed her daughter. Jesus always saw beyond the surface. He knows what is in the heart of each one of us. He sees us not as focus groups, but as persons.

A couple weeks ago a national study tried to lump Catholic women together in a group. The Guttmacher study of some 1000 women who had abortions, said 29% of the abortions were procured by Catholic women. And then they attempted to make a connection between that statistic and the Church's teaching on birth control.

However they downplayed some facts from their own study. A woman who describes herself as religious, that is who practices her faith, whether Protestant or Catholic, is only 25% as likely to seek an abortion as the average. There is a big difference between a cultural Catholic and a practicing Catholic. To use a personal comparison: I might sometimes say I am a "Croatian" because my mom's parents came from that country, but if I meet a real Croatian, I recognize a huge difference.

It is similar between those who call themselves "Catholic" and those who are living and breathing their faith. Now, we don't reject a cultural Catholic, in fact, we're glad they acknowledge their baptism, but we want them to return to the *full* practice of their faith and start attending Mass; that makes all the difference.

A deep relation to Jesus through the Church he founded is what we offer. As he did for the daughter of the Canaanite, Jesus can free us. Jesus did not come to condemn, but to save. That applies even in the case of abortion. Some people have heard that abortion is one of the very few sins that incur automatic excommunication. That is to underscore its seriousness—the taking of an innocent human life. However, you must also know the priest has authority to lift that excommunication in the sacrament of confession. What is more, in that sacrament Jesus gives not only his forgiveness, but deep healing.

Since my return from Peru, I have seen how many of our young people, men as well as women, need that healing. Obviously not just for abortion, but a range of sins which affect our souls as was the case of that young woman gripped by a demon.

Part of the orientation we want to give to our young people is an understanding of their sexuality. Why God created us male and female. Our society is in deep trouble because we have lost that orientation. The terrible plague of abortion which I referred to is one symptom. But I want to be clear. The solution to abortion is not more birth control. In that same Guttmacher study *57% of the women who had abortions were using birth control in the month before they got pregnant.*

Those of us who are older can remember when the birth control pill was first introduced in the late 50's. It was presented as the solution to all our biggest problems: overpopulation, unwanted pregnancies, abortions, child abuse, large unhappy families, and above all marital tension between husband and wife. After 35 years of widespread use of the birth control pill and other forms of artificial contraception, I believe we are ready to ask: Is birth control really the solution or is it the problem?

An amazing article came out last month in U.S. News and World Report, not exactly a Catholic magazine. Lionel Tiger who is an evolutionary anthropologist asked why there has been so much family breakdown, male irresponsibility, single parents and abortion since the 1960's. He says the main reason is the massive use of the birth control pill.

There is an alternative. I had the opportunity to take the Creighton University course on Natural Family Planning which is offered to doctors, nurses, clergy and NFP practitioners. There have been tremendous advances in Natural Family Planning since the 60s. I hope to say more about that in the future and certainly to share it with our engaged couples and any young married couples. I have also contacted some doctors, women gynecologists right here in Seattle who are willing to work with couples on using natural methods.

When I was in Peru I worked with a married couple and an obstetrician to teach Natural Family Planning. Some 100 couples participated. We also offered a class for young adults, singles, who wanted to be instructors or promoters. Not only young women, but young men attended. Of course the boys could not keep a personal chart as the girls could. So they asked their moms if they could do a chart for them. The course lasted six months and when it was over I asked one of the boys what he had learned. He said to me, "Father, I learned respect for women."

That is what our society needs—and that is what Natural Family Planning promotes. I am convinced that Jesus Christ and the teachings of the Church he founded are the solution to the problems of our society—and our own deepest personal needs.

Like the Canaanite woman we come to Jesus with our needs, with the needs of those we love. If we had her humility, we would also hear Jesus loving words, "Your faith is great. Your prayer is granted."

Seek and You Shall Find: The Beauty of Humanae Vitae

By Father McLean Cummings
Diocese of Baltimore, On Assignment with
Aid to Russia

The Church is a mother to her children, and she will not give them evil gifts. When the People of God cry out: "Show us Jesus Christ! Preach the Gospel to us! Tell us how to attain eternal life," the Church responds, bolstered by her charism of infallibility, with the authentic Gospel entrusted to her by Christ himself. Her goal, like any mother's, is only that her children be happy and fulfilled. Our Lord said: *Ask and you will receive that your joy may be full.* (Jn 16:24) He sought to impose no useless burdens on his disciples, but only a light burden and a sweet yoke. Holy Mother Church does not wish to bind up unnecessary burdens either, as the Pharisees did, but she will preach the whole truth, *in season and out of season*.

This weekend the Church celebrates the 30th anniversary of a landmark encyclical letter, written by Paul VI, on the regulation of procreation. This document, known as *Humanae Vitae*, affirmed that God, in his wisdom, arranged that man and woman should cooperate through an act of love with the creation of each new human being. If spouses, consciously and freely, do anything to frustrate the life-giving potential of their married love (that is, by contraception or sterilization), they sin gravely. Today we celebrate the courage of Paul VI in reminding the world of this truth, thanking God for his enlightenment of the Church on this matter. We also pray for the many Catholics who have failed to understand or accept this essential element of the Church's moral doctrine. Many have suspected their mother of giving them a snake when they asked for a fish. Let us pray for these wayward children that the Father give them the Holy Spirit as he has generously promised to do for all who ask!

At the beginning of the 20th century there was nearly unanimous agreement by religious and civil leaders that contraception was a moral and social evil. In 1930 the Anglican church…wavered and allowed contraception in certain cases. Pius XI reacted immediately with a strong affirmation of the sanctity of marriage, denouncing contraception as directly opposed to it. In the 1960's, Paul VI, while always affirming that he would never consider revising Pius XI's position, undertook a study to see if the new hormonal pills were of a different ethical nature than the contraceptive practices condemned throughout the history of the Church. He declared, 30 years ago yesterday, that they were essentially the same, that is, equally opposed to the sanctity of marriage and the good of the spouses. In so doing, Pope Paul VI opened up for the Church a splendid era of clearer theological understanding of marriage and family and great strides in the development of natural methods of regulating procreation.

It is not possible, of course, nor appropriate to try to explain now the many theological, psychological, social and medical reasons which combine in a sort of symphony to show that Paul VI was indeed speaking on behalf of the Creator and Redeemer of Life when he reaffirmed the unlawfulness of contraception. Rather than present arguments, let us consider the fruit that has come from the general acceptance of contraception, for from its fruits we can know the tree.

The first bad fruit that Paul VI predicted in his letter was promiscuity. Certainly, the last 30 years have seen a dramatic increase in that. Suffice to point out that there is a billboard on highway 895, advertising paternity testing, that asks "Who is the Daddy?" This would have been unthinkable in 1968, but we are not outraged, because we have grown so dulled and deadened by slow increases of immorality.

A related bad fruit is divorce. As soon as the Anglicans allowed contraception in 1930, the divorce rate among Protestants began to rise. A few decades later, when Catholics began to use contraception in significant numbers, the divorce rate among us began to rise, too. Why? The couple cuts itself off from God, the source of love. The man begins to objectify his wife. Her dignity as a woman, the giver of life, is devalued. She feels unloved, and distance between them grows. An authority on love, Mother Teresa, explains: "In destroying the power of giving life or loving through contraception, a husband or wife is doing something to self. This turns the attention to self, and so it destroys the gift of love in him and her. In loving, the husband and wife turn the attention to each other, as happens in Natural Family Planning, and not to self, as happens in contraception."

Mother Teresa continues, mentioning the third bad fruit of contraception. "Once that loving is destroyed by contraception, abortion follows very easily. That's why I never give a child [up for adoption] to a family that has used contraception, because if the mother has destroyed the power of loving, how will she love my child?" And so it is that contraception leads not only to divorce but also abortion. Our present Pope affirms, "[T]he popularization of artificial contraception leads to abortion, for both lie—though at different levels—on the same line of fear of the child, rejection of life, lack of respect for the act or the fruit of the union, such as it is established between man and woman by the creator of nature." Technology has now blurred the distinction further so that many products marketed and used as contraceptives actually work by killing newly conceived babies before they can implant. In fact there are many more abortions caused imperceptibly by what is called "contraception" than by surgical means. Thus, tragically, many Catholics have become active cooperators in the culture of death.

Yet there is hope. There are some who have struggled, in Pope Paul VI's words, "against the tide of thought and opinion in a world of paganized behavior." As the Lord surveys the Sodom of our time, he may be able to find "ten just men" amongst it. There are some brave and generous Christians who will always be "the soul of the world," a witness of authentic love in a culture of hedonism and death.

We must convince the world that God has not given his children, through Paul VI, a scorpion when they asked for an egg. He knows what is good for us; he made us. The Church's stand on contraception is not a cold, useless, man-made rule. Rather, *Humanae Vitae* is part of the Gospel law of liberty; it liberates couples for authentic Christian love. It is possible and joyful to obey for those who *have been raised with [Christ] through their belief in the power of God.* Let no one think that he cannot fulfill the demands of an authentically human life. As John Paul II encouraged some Indonesian bishops: "Let us never fear that the challenge is too great for our people. They were redeemed by the precious blood of Christ. They are his people...It is he, Jesus Christ, who will continue to give the grace to his people to meet the requirements of his word...what is impossible with man is possible with God." (AAS 71, 1979, p. 1423)

What remains for us is to be what we are: a new creation, a people set apart: "*Be not conformed to this world, but be transformed by the renewal of your mind,*" said St. Paul. If you cannot see the beauty of *Humanae Vitae*: *seek and you shall find.* If you cannot imagine ever being able to live it: *ask and you shall receive.* Never think you have no alternative to sin, but *knock and the door will be opened to you.*

Children Make Us More Human

By Father Brian Doerr
Director of Vocations, Diocese of Lafayette, Indiana

For many years now, I have been troubled by the manner in which people sometimes enter a restaurant and until recently, I have never understood why. Have you ever noticed what occurs if you happen to park in a restaurant parking lot while another car simultaneously does the same? You have experienced this: the driver of the other car, and his or her party, will have the car unloaded and the party will, without looking at you, walk quickly, while consciously maneuvering to arrive at the restaurant door before you. Once they have reached the door, they ease a bit and casually walk in…before you, of course. Time and time again, I have seen this occur.

The object of the game is getting into the restaurant before the other people so you do not have to wait for a table and can receive your food before everyone else. There is lacking in this, a sense of etiquette, decorum or decency. And why does this "trivial little matter" bother me? Just recently I linked this with a larger trend in our culture, and now I see it as a symptom of something much greater.

We have, as a culture and as an economic system, developed a frightening sense of competition. The people who live in our world are in a desperate mode of heightened rivalry. Why can a man not rush to the door of a restaurant and hold the door for his fellow citizens and allow them to pass first? The answer: because he is in *competition* with them and he must be careful not to loose his place. Competition is no longer confined to sports or the marketplace. Needless to say, the United States has become quite good at competing. As a nation, we compete to consume a disproportionately large share of the world's natural resources.

As individuals, we compete to make more money in order to acquire a greater portion of goods and services. We compete with each other for fame and prestige. We compete with the clothes we purchase and the make-up we wear. We compete to have the best technological equipment, the best automobiles, and the best and largest houses. Simply watch advertisements with a critical eye and see how marketers are manipulating us to compete against one another.

No longer do we see our neighbor as a brother or sister made in the image and likeness of God to be respected and treated with dignity; he or she is a competitor—competing to consume or steal what we have acquired or want to acquire. The implications run deep. Our Holy Father, the defender of all human life, reminds us that:

> Despite their differences of nature and moral gravity, contraception and abortion are often closely connected, as fruits of the same tree. It is true that in many cases contraception and even abortion are practiced under the pressure of real life difficulties, which nonetheless can never exonerate from striving to observe God's law fully. Still, in very many other instances such practices are rooted in a hedonistic mentality unwilling to accept responsibility in matters of sexuality, and they imply a self-centered concept of freedom, *which regards procreation as an obstacle to personal fulfillment*. The life which could result from a sexual encounter thus becomes an enemy to be avoided at all costs, and abortion becomes the only possible decisive response to failed contraception (EV 13).

Rather than embracing the gift of the unborn child, we have come, as a culture, to see the child as a competitor—both on the national level as well as the personal level—"an obstacle to personal fulfillment."

One of the most outspoken promoters of abortion throughout the world has used the United Nations to promote abortion because, as she claims, the world does not have the resources to sustain its population growth. She, and others from our country, have targeted third world countries in particular because we do not want "those people" to consume "our resources." Yet she lives in, not one, but two mansions: one in California and one in Montana. And we wonder, if the world cannot sustain such a great population because of its limited resources, why does she not remove herself from her mansions and freely share the resources she selfishly consumes? Because people have become competitors. She is unwilling to allow life as life may mean the loss of her "things."

Furthermore, if we look past the continuous lies and deceit of the pro-death lobby, we can see on the personal level that the unwanted child is unconsciously perceived as a competitor to his/her own parents. The child competes against the mother and father's own desires, material goods, career plans, financial resources, and personal agendas. The killing of over seven thousand weak and defenseless human beings every day because they compete against our own self-centered desires is a crime beyond reckoning.

In addition, children are no longer considered miraculous gifts of God, they have become products. If wanted, these products can be purchased (custom ordered) through artificial reproduction or, if unwanted, they can be aborted or prevented by contraception. A wise man, David C. Stolinsky in an article entitled, "*A Nation of Narcissists?*" quipped, "Narcissists view their children the way they view their BMW—prized possessions to be shown off. Like the BMW, the kids are pampered but cared for by others, from nannies to daycare providers to teachers, not to mention math tutors and soccer coaches. Many of the joys and pains of having kids are experienced by others. And kids are under pressure to get into the best schools, to provide more grounds for boasting, and to make more money (*New Oxford Review*, June 2002)."

Is it not time to heed the voice of St. Elizabeth Anne Seton who said, "live simply, that others might live"? Is it not time we cease looking at our brothers and sisters and sons and daughters as competitors for our resources or products to own, and begin to love them as we love ourselves—just as Jesus taught us?

The mystery of parenthood is not difficult to discern. A child comes into our life to crush our selfishness and makes us more human—loving, generous, patient, kind and selfless humans. When the baby begins to cry at 3 AM, a parent learns selflessness, just as I learn selflessness when someone is dying at the hospital at 3 AM. Parents learn selflessness when their six-year-old wants him or her to read her a book, just as I learn selflessness when a teenager wants to go to Confession after I've already heard two hours of confessions. And parents learn selflessness when money must be saved for college or for insurance for the children, just as I learn selflessness when financially limited by my attempt to live simply like Jesus.

I learned a valuable lesson in my last parish. Every Sunday after Mass I was greeted by a man named Doug who was mildly mentally handicapped. Most people today would consider him a drain on society, not contributing to the welfare of the state and, worse, competing for the resources that we desire to consume. Many people like Doug are aborted every day—their parents not willing to subject themselves to the trials of raising a special needs baby for such "little" reward.

Doug, to the shock of his family, had a massive heart attack and died suddenly. It was tremendously difficult for his family and friends and the day of the funeral saw a church packed with people: the largest funeral I had witnessed during my time as a priest. Men and women alike outwardly mourned Doug's passing.

The conclusion is not hard to draw. In the eyes of the world, Doug did nothing but consume our precious little resources. But if Doug, indeed, contributed nothing to our culture, our economy, or our society, he certainly taught a huge number of people how to love. In a sense, he was an apostle of love, and the day he was buried, his disciples came in large numbers to say good-bye.

We can learn from Doug that all people are made in God's image and have infinite value and to compete against our brother or sister is to reject all that Christ Jesus revealed to us. As an old Dominican priest once impressed upon me, "be generous with God," he whispered as if telling a secret, "and he will be generous with you." No better way to summarize the calling of parents, priests or any worthwhile vocation.

Revisiting Humanae Vitae
By Most Reverend John F. Donoghue, DD
Archbishop of Atlanta

Closing of the Conference on *Humanae Vitae*

July 21, 2001

Dear Friends in Christ,

Thirty-three years ago, this month, the birth of *Humanae Vitae*, Pope Paul VI's definitive encyclical on the transmission of human life, was not accomplished without pain and suffering. I remember well the travails that our Mother, the Church, went through as this child of wisdom made its way into a world already set on a course of opposition and rejection.

I was Chancellor of the Archdiocese of Washington at the time, and as events unfolded within a few days, I realized that the Church, both the faithful and the clergy, and that I myself, would forever be changed by the publication of this momentous and decisive document.

For it was no surprise, but still a great disappointment, when within a day of the publication of *Humanae Vitae*, more than sixty priests of the Archdiocese of Washington, announced, by publishing it in the *Washington Post*, their opposition to the teachings of the Holy Father, of the Church, of the Magisterium, and we must believe, of the Holy Spirit.

The Cardinal Archbishop of Washington, Patrick O'Boyle, with no happiness about it, called me into his office, and said, "We cannot let this go by. Call every one of the priests named in the protest. Tell them I am suspending their faculties to celebrate the Sacraments, and let them know that I am ready and anxious to speak with each of them individually."

It was undoubtedly one of the hardest moments he had ever faced, and in assisting him at this difficult moment, it was also a moment in time that changed me—for it left upon me the scars of battle, scars we must and will win, if we engage to defend the Church against her opponents, and if we strive to win back, those who have set themselves against the Church and her God-given teachings.

The Church struggles still with the difficulties of putting *Humanae Vitae* into practice, and part of the reason we are here is to pray for the guidance of the Holy Spirit as we attempt, in our own time, to make this teaching a more accepted and vital part of the Church's ongoing life and mission.

But even Pope Paul VI, in his prophetic wisdom, possibly did not see all the trends, all the movements, all the individual perversities that were to be raised against the sanctity of life in the years since he spoke so forcefully against the comparatively simple sin of artificial contraception.

The evolving disregard for the conception and generation of life, has been, in large part, responsible for even more outrageous acts against life in other phases of its existence. Abortion and euthanasia, the front and back doors of the house of the culture of death, have now opened to reveal rooms of more insidious evil, harbored between these two portals of hell. Eugenics, genetic engineering, cloning, embryonic stem cell research; these are the inevitable progeny of man's arrogant assumption of the management of life, which began with the pro-contraception movements.

Where can it lead from here? We can only wonder, and acknowledge the aptness of the old prayer, which describes the "wickedness and snares of the devil," and admit that the genius of man, when turned to evil, is indeed amazing, and true to the nature of original sin, diabolical as well.

But for the Church, for Catholics, for all spouses who live in the family of the Church, and who wish to make peace with their consciences, *Humanae Vitae* is far more than a prophecy and a recollection of what could and what did go wrong. *Humane Vitae* is in fact, the roadmap to marital sanctity and marital stability—and more—it is the map which will ultimately lead to a better world, at least for those who follow its guiding lights.

In this Sunday's Gospel, we hear of a decisive moment in the lives of our Lord's disciples, not a moment of conflict limited to Mary and Martha, not just our Lord's solution to the anger of Martha and perhaps the satisfaction of Mary, but a moment of decision for all Christians. Which is to be the most important focus in life—living a life in service to goodness, or living a life in service to the Lord? The two seem close, and in some cases, seem to be the same thing. But they are not. Ethical people are good people—and we get along with them, respect them, and live with them in peace. But Christians are people who are ethical *because they are the Lord's*. The goodness which brings salvation comes from devotion to the Lord. Goodness in and of itself saves no one. Christ did not say, "Do good, and that will take care of your sins." Christ said, *"You shall love the Lord your God with all your heart, with all your soul and with all your mind...*

and love your neighbor as yourself." It is clear that love of God must come first, and then the rest will follow.

Such a moment of decision is reflected in the teachings of *Humanae Vitae*. Plenty of seemingly responsible husbands and wives decide, on their own, that for the good of everyone involved, they must limit the number of lives they will conceive, and that the easiest, most practical way of doing this is by artificial contraception, the unnatural interruption of the act of conception. To do this is to commit the fault of Martha—to put convenience, to put material considerations, to put comfort above the first duty of marriage, which is, to love and serve God by doing His will. And His will, as expressed by the Church, under the guidance of the Holy Spirit, is not to interfere unnaturally with the generation of life. *Humanae Vitae* is the blueprint for incorporating the will of God into the life of Christian marriage. And the fruits of such obedience are beautifully laid out by Pope Paul VI, when he writes:

> …discipline imbues love with a deeper human meaning. Although self-control requires continuous effort, it also helps the spouses become strong in virtue and makes them rich with spiritual goods. And this virtue fosters the fruits of tranquility and peace in the home and helps in the solving of difficulties of other kinds. It aids spouses in becoming more tender with each other and more attentive to each other. It assists them in dispelling that inordinate self-love that is opposed to true charity. It strengthens in them an awareness of their responsibilities. And finally it provides parents with a sure and efficacious authority for educating their children. As their children advance through life they will come to a correct appreciation of the true goods of man and employ peacefully and properly the powers of their mind and senses.

Dear friends, these are beautiful promises, but they are promises based on the truth of God. Therefore, they can and do come true, not without difficulty, as Pope Paul reminds us, nor "without the help of God, who upholds and strengthens the good will of men."

May this conference, may the efforts of all who have joined in planning and attending it, may the example that you, our Catholic husbands and wives, set by the way you live your own marriages, and above all, may the help of God, we constantly implore, reinvigorate in our local Church an awareness and appreciation for the great gift of *Humanae Vitae*, Pope Paul VI's finest and most enduring effort on behalf of the People of God, the Holy Catholic Church.

And may the fruits of tranquility and peace, harvested in your hearts and your homes, by surrendering to the sharp sweetness of God's law, bring new life, new compassion, and new wisdom to the world around us.

This we pray, in our Lord's name. Amen.

Reprinted with permission, Godsplanforlife.com.

God's Plan for Human Life
By Fr. Matthew Habiger, O.S.B., PhD
St. Benedict's Abbey, Atchison, Kansas

Introduction

We are now in the first Easter Season of the New Millennium. After the great Jubilee Year of grace, we are still reflecting upon the significance of Easter and all that God has done for us through the life, death and resurrection of His Son. We know that remarkable things lie in store for us. With six billion people alive today, and with the advantages of education, science, and technology, we have every reason to believe that the 21st Century will either be a time of heightened religious experience or a time of great peril.

God's Plan for Human Life Reaffirmed by Easter

The events of Holy Week and Easter reaffirm God's original plan for us. Jesus came into the world to overcome the damage caused by our sin, the damage caused by our choosing evil over goodness, by preferring our ways over God's ways. We had fallen into a pit out of which we were unable to climb. This necessitated that the Son of God Himself come into our world as one of us, that He teach us how to live this life well, that is, to live the Christian life, and eventually that He lay down His life for us. Remember, Jesus died for our sins once and forever. Christ's body was important for him in His Resurrection and in our Redemption. This tells us something about the importance of our own bodies.

We Are Bodied Persons

As human beings, we need to understand our condition as a person who has a body. Our bodies are very important. By means of our body, we are present to the world, and the world is present to us. There was never a time when we were absent from our bodies. Our bodies have a definite life cycle which everyone experiences.

We also know that our bodies are gifts to us from God, just as is human life and good health. We are expected to understand our bodies, our bodied condition as a bodied person. We must learn how to respect our bodies and cooperate in allowing our bodies to assist us in living our lives in this world well. We are talking here about God's plan for human life, human love, and human family.

An Analogy: The Gift of Taste and Eating

We usually take good health for granted, and then begin to abuse it. Take, for example, the gift of taste and eating. We know that we must eat in order to nourish our bodies. Eating is also a very social event. Mealtimes are times when families and friends come together to strengthen their bondedness. Tasty, succulent food enhances the meal.

But if the pleasure of eating becomes an end in itself, if we eat just for the sake of eating, then very soon we do real damage to ourselves and to our bodies. Obesity results, in most cases, from abuses of the body. Wealthy nations have a real problem with obesity. God's plan for eating is that we eat a well-balanced diet and use moderation. Eat for a purpose; don't make the purpose of life mere eating.

The Gift of Fertility and Human Sexuality

In a similar way God has a plan for our fertility and human sexuality. It is important to remember that our bodies and all that they contain are God's gift to us. We had nothing to do with the designing of our bodies; it was strictly God's plan. Parents have relatively little to contribute to the essential physical design of their child's body.

God most assuredly has a plan for our fertility and human sexuality. It is a very good plan. As intelligent and responsible human persons, we are able to know God's plan, to appreciate its goodness, and then to freely choose to live by it.

God's plan includes allowing us to be co-creators with Him, and to provide a means of close bonding between a husband and wife. Although our sexuality provides great pleasure, pleasure is a "companion good" and not the chief focus. Like eating, or drinking, or any other physical activity, sex can be abused. And if the conception of a new human person is involved, a person endowed with our own human dignity, then terrible harm can be done. If a person can be hurt badly by being used as an object for someone's gratification, then there is nothing trivial about sexual behavior.

Our world is very confused about God's plan for fertility and human sexuality. Some people think that they can make up their own rules and define sex anyway they want. It is just a matter of preference or choice. Something like ordering items from a menu in a restaurant. They think this, despite the fact that the human person is the only thing God created for its own sake. "In His own image He made them male and female" (Gen 1:26). Only a person lives forever. Only a person can love and be loved. Only for the sake of a person with such dignity would God send His only Son into the world to atone for our sins by his own suffering and death.

God's Plan for Love, Life and Family=Chastity

My brothers and sisters, as we move into the new century we are encouraged to be a people of hope and expectation. We know that we have the potential of doing great good. We know that we have received many blessings from God, and that He expects great things from us—even difficult things.

We know that most of the problems on this earth are of our own making, and that we can both correct what is wrong and build up what is good and helpful to others. This requires that we learn God's plan for love, life and the family. It means the total gift of self by a man to his wife, and the total gift of self by a woman to her husband. This means no sex before marriage, and total fidelity within marriage. It means no abortion, sterilization, or contraception. It means acquiring the virtue of chastity.

St. John Chrysostom suggests that young husbands should say to their wives: "I have taken you in my arms, and I love you, and I prefer you to my life itself…I place your love above all things, and nothing would be more bitter or painful to me than to be of a different mind than you" (CCC 2346).

Pope John Paul II speaks of fertility as part of mutual self-gift and enhancing the dignity of the human person: "The innate language (of the marital embrace) expresses the total reciprocal self-giving of husband and wife. Contraception is an objectively contradictory language, namely, that of not giving oneself totally to the other. This leads not only to a positive refusal to be open to life but also to a falsification of the inner truth of conjugal love, which is called upon to give itself in personal totality" (FC 32, CCC 2370).

God wants what is best for His sons and daughters. He never asks the impossible—just the plain difficult. Chastity is a difficult virtue; it always has been. Chastity always benefits our marriages, our families, and the wider culture. The absence of chastity always brings great harm and misery to everyone it affects.

I encourage you, at the dawn of a new century and the new millennium, read the encyclical *Humanae Vitae* It has a clear formula for happiness and well being for everyone.

Easter means that we are called to be a people of hope and expectation. We have every right to be optimistic about the future. Indeed, we can be victorious in the struggle between good and evil. We can live a life pleasing to God and beneficial to ourselves. We can keep the Commandments and live the Christian life. This means everyone, since God's call to holiness is universal. His call to holiness is given to everyone, to every culture and to every walk of life. In short, we are all called to become saints, a people who are very close to God.

Reprinted with permission, Godsplanforlife.com

Trinity Sunday Homily
By Father Matthew Habiger, O.S.B., PhD
St. Benedict's Abbey, Atchison, Kansas

26 May 2002

This is Trinity Sunday. Following Ascension Thursday and Pentecost, it brings together the involvement of the Father, the Son, and the Holy Spirit in our salvation. Remember: all three persons of the Blessed Trinity are involved with us, and we with them.

God is the most profound of all mysteries. He is the creator of the entire universe, all that exists. He created all the angels. He created the human race, beginning with our first parents, Adam and Eve. God is one. Christianity is monotheistic, not polytheistic. But within the one Godhead there are three persons. Three persons in one God. In his full grandeur and complexity, God exceeds our limited vision and our poor understanding. But God has given us ways and means of knowing something about Him. The Father sent His Son among us as one of us. Jesus, in turn, taught us about the Father. And now the Holy Spirit helps us understand the full meaning of Jesus' words.

One very good way to explain the Holy Trinity today is to think of a *communion of persons*. We know something about what it means to enter into a communion with another person. We make the gift of ourselves to a friend, and accept the gift of our friend to us. There is a sharing of hearts, of minds, of wills, of our very person. Marriage, as God designed it, is the clearest example of this: the husband makes the total gift of himself to his spouse. She accepts his gift, and then offers the total gift of herself to him. And he receives her, appreciating the rich significance of the gift of her person to him, a communion of persons.

Apply this now to God. Among the three persons of God, there is a total communion of love and life. The love of the Father and the Son issues forth in the person of the Holy Spirit. The love, life, and creative energy among these three divine persons become one dynamic communion, one God: a communion of three persons in one God.

The Vatican II document, *Gaudium et Spes*, speaks about God's design for the communitarian nature of the human vocation: "The Lord Jesus, when praying to the Father 'that they may all be one...even as we are one' (Jn 17:21-2), has opened up new horizons closed to human reason by indicating that there is a certain similarity between the union existing among the divine persons and the union of God's children in truth and love It follows, then, that if human beings are the only creatures on earth that God has wanted for their own sake, they can fully discover their true selves only in sincere self-giving" (24).

My brothers and sisters, I want to relate this "communion of persons," and this "making the gift of self" to *our situation in these times.* The recent sex scandals by some clergy are forcing us to re-examine God's plan for us as bodied persons. We recall that God alone designed human nature, and that He alone designs the moral order. He alone determines what is right and what is wrong.

I am going to talk about God's plan for human love and life, about chastity, and about *violations against God's plan, especially contraception and sterilization.* You probably have not heard these topics discussed before from this pulpit, or for that matter from other pulpits. And for that we priests are guilty in the negligence of our duty to teach clearly God's plan for human love and human life. I ask you now to forgive us our negligence in performing our duties.

This is a time for all of us to return to the basics about our sexuality, about the fact that we are bodied persons. The natural attraction between a man and a woman (Adam and Eve), the desire to become "one flesh" is good and noble. But this desire must be expressed according to God's design for human love and life. The only proper place for sex is in marriage. Outside of marriage sex is wrong and sinful. It violates God's plan for human love. Similarly, within marriage, God also has a plan. That plan calls for making the total gift of self from one spouse to another, a total sharing of one's self with one's spouse, a communion of persons. This sharing *includes our fertility.* Sex and fertility go together. We cannot hold back part of the gift and pretend we are giving and receiving the full gift of self.

When we reflect upon the nature of conjugal love, we soon realize that it is *both unitive* (love-giving) *and procreative* (life-giving). True love is always life-giving in one way or another. I am a celibate, but my love for you and for others is always life-giving. Contraception and sterilization always go wrong by withdrawing the total gift of self, by attacking the goodness of our fertility and considering it something evil to be destroyed, by refusing to be open to the gift of a new life.

The encyclical *Humanae Vitae* predicted the tragic results of widespread contraception: a weakening of moral discipline; a trivialization of human sexuality; the demeaning of women; marital infidelity; state sponsored programs of population control; the introduction of legalized abortion and euthanasia, the idea of unlimited dominion over one's body and life as seen now in genetic manipulation and embryo experimentation.

The teaching of *Humanae Vitae* honors married love, promotes the dignity of women, and helps couples grow in understanding the truth of their particular path to holiness. It is also a response to contemporary society's temptation to reduce life to a commodity.

My brothers and sisters, on this feast of the Blessed Trinity, I encourage you to learn more about God's wonderful plan for human life and human love, about marriage and family. Learn why men and women are the only creatures on earth God wanted for their own sake, and why we can fully discover our true selves only in sincere self-giving.

I encourage you to get a copy of *Humanae Vitae* and study it. It is a very clear statement of God's plan for human life and human love. I encourage you to learn about Natural Family Planning (NFP), God's way and nature's way of exercising responsible parenthood. NFP helps couples discover something of the richness of their being bodied persons, made "in the image and likeness of God."

Reprinted with permission, Godsplanforlife.com.

The Church's Moral Teaching on Contraception, Part 1

By Father Anthony Kopp, O Praem
St. Michael's Abbey, Norbertine Fathers of Orange County

This is the first homily of a three-part series given by Fr. Kopp, O Praem, recorded at St. Kilian Church, Mission Viejo, CA.

Jesus gives a very stern warning this morning when He says that if he refuses to listen even to the Church then treat him as you would a gentile or tax collector. In other words Jesus was telling us if we refuse to listen to his Church, then we're in big trouble. There is one particular moral issue in which surveys, at least, show that many Catholics don't think or act in accordance with the teaching of the Church and that is rather unfortunate indeed. As a priest, of course, following the warning given by the prophet of today's first reading, I have to warn you that on this particular moral issue, many Catholics are off base. They are doing what is wrong and wicked.

Now, what is this moral issue? Probably a lot of you think Father is going to talk about abortion. No, I am not. I am going to talk about an issue which is more fundamental than that, which is morally evil, which opens the door to abortion in our country. It is a moral issue which I think is probably the most important issue today. This evil has done more to undermine our society and our Church than any other. It is so important, in fact that I am going to devote many homilies in a row to this topic. So by now you are probably wondering what is this moral issue.

Well, to introduce it I want to give a little quiz. It is a 3-question true/false quiz. Just answer on your own to yourself; don't shout out the answer.

No Christian church ever accepted contraception as morally permissible before 1930. Is that true or false?

A Protestant legislature, for a largely Protestant America, passed the anti-contraceptive laws of 19th century America, true or false?

The leaders of the Protestant Reformation were strongly opposed to unnatural forms of birth control, true or false?

Let's be honest. How many answered "true" to all 3 of those? That is correct, all 3 are true. It is a historical fact that no Christian church accepted contraception before 1930. In fact, up until 1930 every Christian church strongly condemned the use of unnatural forms of birth control. It was only in 1930 that the Lambeth Conference of the Anglican Church first allowed the use of such things in certain select cases. It is a historical fact in the last century, our Protestant legislatures passed laws which prohibited, under penalty of law, the purchase and manufacture or even possession of contraceptive devices. It was against the law. Finally the leaders of the Protestant Reformation and in particular, Martin Luther, strongly condemned the use of unnatural forms of birth control. So, we see that at least for nineteen hundred and thirty years of Christianity, contraception was condemned by all Christians and was seen as a great evil.

Now why did Christians teach that, and why does the Catholic Church today continue to teach that the use of unnatural forms of birth control is a grave moral evil? It is, in fact, a grave sin. Why does the Church teach that? Well, because of what God has revealed—and today in the remaining part of this homily, I want to sketch out to you where exactly God speaks to us about this issue.

Well, first of all, we need to keep in mind what God teaches us about human life and the value of human life, and His desire to see human life brought into this world. First, you may recall way back in the Book of Genesis, the very first chapter after God has created Adam and Eve, God gave them a command which is recorded in the first chapter and 28th verse of Genesis. God says this to Adam and Eve. God blessed them, saying, "be fertile and multiply, fill the earth and subdue it." Be fertile and multiply, and if you read the 150 psalms, frequently God tells us there, that, children are His gifts. They are something to be treasured. For example, in Psalm 127 v. 3, God says this, "Behold sons and daughters are a gift from the Lord. The fruit of the womb is a reward." In other words, children are a blessing. Now we need to keep this in mind because obviously we are living in a society that does not promote such a view. In fact, our Holy Father has told us over and over again that we are living, very sadly, in a culture of death, a society that promotes death.

Just yesterday I was reading about a Supreme Court decision in my home state of Wisconsin. Wisconsin is now the first state that has passed a law that requires a woman to have a 24-hour waiting period before she has an abortion. And the law in the state of Wisconsin says that a woman must be given an opportunity when she goes to an abortion clinic to hear the heartbeat of her unborn child. They have to allow her to hear that heartbeat, then give her time to make her decision. Well, pro-abortionists took that to the Supreme Court of Wisconsin, saying that was some sort of coercive pro-life conspiracy to eliminate abortions. That is ridiculous of course, but it shows just how far we have come now, in our pro-death mentality, that we seem to, for whatever reason, favor death over life.

So we see that God wants us to be generous in bringing human life into this world and it is a gift from Him. But we might ask a question then. Did God say anything in particular about the use of unnatural means of birth control? Is there any mention in the Sacred Scripture? The answer is yes, there is. And once again we find it in the Book of Genesis, Ch. 38. Now I need to give you a little background material before I read this account to you. In the Old Testament there was a particular law, which stated that if a man took a wife and then the man died before any children were born, that the brother of that man should take his wife, a widow, and bear children with her and that those children would then be attributed to the man who had died. That was the law in the Old Testament. In this particular case we see in chapter 38, a man named Er has taken a woman named Tamar as his wife and before they have any children, Er dies. And so, therefore, Judah, who is the father of Er says to his son Onan, that he must take Tamar to be his wife, and have children which must be attributed to Er. And then the story goes like this.

"Onan, however, knew that the descendants would not be counted as his, they would be counted as his brother Er's. So whenever he had relations with his brother's widow, Tamar, he wasted his seed on the ground to avoid contributing offspring for his brother."

Notice that he wasted his seed on the ground. What he did greatly offended the Lord and the Lord took his life. As punishment for that sin, the unnatural act that Onan was committing, God took his life. God saw it as a serious moral evil and therefore in punishment for that sin, God took the life of Onan. And it is very interesting to know—I don't think some of you might be aware of this—up until recently in the history of the Church, unnatural forms of birth control were called what? - acts of Onanism. Why? Because of this account right here in the Book of Genesis; this unnatural act of birth control practiced by Onan. The root for that word "Onanism" is found right here in this verse. It shows us clearly what God finds unfavorable—that God is strongly opposed to this particular act, this unnatural act of birth control.

Now in modern times, when the push is to contracept, certain scripture scholars have tried to reinterpret this passage saying that Onan was not punished by God for wasting his seed, but that he was punished because he was not open to his obligation to Tamar. However, as it is recorded in Deuteronomy 25, the punishment for not fulfilling the law is not death, but rather embarrassment in front of the community. So it shows us that God was attaching a special punishment to the sin of Onan, because that particular act was abominable in his sight. And of course that has been the interpretation from the Church from the very beginning: that God is very displeased with unnatural forms of birth control.

We might ask ourselves, is there any reference to birth control in the New Testament? Some scripture scholars think that there is. In Revelation 21:8, God says this: "But as for cowards, the unfaithful, the depraved, murderers, the unchaste, sorcerers, idol worshippers, and deceivers of every sort, their lot is in the burning pool of fire and sulfur, which is the second death." In other words God is telling us here that if we practice these things and don't repent, that hell will be our lot for all eternity. Now if you were listening really closely there, of course you didn't hear the word "contraception" or anything that sounded like it. Well, the word that could be used for "contraception" is the word "sorcery." That's because in the original Greek, the word that is used is "pharmaceia", which sounds like our English word "pharmacy" or "pharmaceutical." It is thought by some Scripture scholars that what's being referred to here is the first century practice of contraception. You see, contraception goes way back. It is not just something from the 20th century. It goes all the way back to the time of Christ, even before. In those days women would concoct certain potions or certain herbs together, which they would drink, thinking that they would cause either a miscarriage or prevent conception. You see, that sort of thing was going on in those days and some Scripture scholars believe that this word "pharmaceia" or "sorcery", is referring to that practice—the practice of concocting those potions to prevent conception or to cause an abortion. So it is thought by some that contraception is discussed even in the New Testament. The bottom line, my brothers and sisters, is that for 2000 years now the Catholic Church, and for 1930 years most Christian churches, have strongly condemned these particular acts, these unnatural forms of birth control. And that's based, in part, on the testimony of God's revelation found in the Sacred Scriptures.

Now there are many today in the Catholic Church that are militating for a change in this teaching, and I would say to them, "Don't you believe as a Catholic, that the Holy Spirit guides the Church? After all, that is a fundamental belief of our faith, that Christ and His Spirit guide the Catholic Church. Well, do you think that the Holy Spirit made a mistake on this issue? Did the Holy Spirit not guide the Church for 2000 years? And all of a sudden we are going to say that while the Holy Spirit guides the Church, we were wrong before, and now the Holy Spirit has changed His mind? Does that make any sense or seem logical? No." The Church, guided by the Holy Spirit, has taught the evil of these acts for 2000 years now and will continue to do so. And the reason is, of course, that God has taught us these things are morally wrong." Now when I teach this to my students in my religion classes, right away the hands will go up and say, "Well, Father, does this mean that if I am going to be a good Catholic mother that I should try to have 25 children? Should I try to have as many children as I possibly can? Is that the teaching of the Church?" Well for the answer to that my brothers and sisters, you will have to wait for the next homily.

Reprinted with permission, Godsplanforlife.com

The Church's Moral Teaching on Contraception, Part 2

By Father Anthony Kopp, O Praem

This is the second homily of a three-part series given by Fr. Anthony Kopp, O Praem, recorded at St. Kilian Church, Mission Viejo, CA.

For a Catholic couple now, how many children are they called by God to bring into this world? I sort of left you with a facetious remark; is a Catholic couple called to bring into this world, let us say for example, 25 children in order to consider themselves a good, holy, Catholic couple? We are going to answer that question today. There will be no better way to answer that than to turn to the teaching of the Church herself, presented in the second Vatican Council 35 years ago. You may recall at that time, 1965, that the final document of the Council was *Gaudium et Spes*, (the "Church in the Modern World.") There is a section in *Gaudium et Spes* on the question of human life—bringing children into this world. I thought it would be a good idea to answer that question by turning to that official teaching of our Church, especially to paragraph 50 and first we read there, the following:

Marriage and married love are by nature ordered to the procreation and education of children. Indeed children are the supreme gift of marriage and greatly contribute to the good of the parents themselves… Married couples should regard it as their proper mission to transmit human life and to educate their children. They should realize that they are thereby cooperating with the love of God, their creator.

Now, let me make a few comments about those sentences which I just read to you from *Gaudium et Spes*. First of all, the Church teaches us—and we saw last time, that this is exactly what God has revealed to us in His Holy Word—that marriage and married love are by nature ordered to bringing children into this world and educating them. Now from time to time when I have taught religion in the past, students have said to me, "Well Father, what if I want to get married, but I don't want to have any children. We are going to, a priori, exclude children from our marriage." Well, I say to them immediately, then you shouldn't get married and you are not ready for marriage. Because the Church teaches us, as God teaches us, one of the primary ends or purposes of marriage is to bring children into this world. So obviously, to enter into marriage to exclude children is wrong. Also the

Council teaches that children are not just *a* gift in marriage, but the **supreme gift of marriage!** I am sure you mothers and fathers have held your children in your arms, after they were born, and you realize this instinctively. The greatest gift of marriage is a new life, a child. When you hold that child, it is quite obvious that this is an expression of love of the couple and what a beautiful gift that is. We read there as well, that children contribute greatly to the good of the parents.

I have two sisters who have children and of course my brothers-in-law as well, and I can see quite clearly, in the past years since they have been married, that they have changed by having children. It does change the couple for the better. Because obviously if you have children you need to grow in love, especially in sacrificial love. You need to sacrifice yourself for your children and of course you need to grow in patience and in other virtues as well. And so bringing children into the world does the couple so much good, especially spiritual good. We read also that the couple has the privilege of cooperating with the love of God, the Creator. As you know, God does not drop down people from heaven. The couple needs to cooperate with God in bringing new life into this world. God will not do it on His own. A husband and wife must cooperate with God, the Creator, in bringing a child into this world. Just think then how close the married couple is to God, the Creator. What a tremendous gift that is, to work so closely with God.

Now, that still doesn't answer the question then, what does God expect with regard to bringing children into this world? How many does He expect? Well the first thing we have to keep in mind is what the Council tells us at the end of this section, where we read, "Among the married couples who thus fulfill their God given mission of bringing children into the world, special mention should be made of those who after prudent reflection and common decision, courageously, undertake the proper upbringing of a large number of children." In other words the Church is teaching us that those Catholic couples who are generous and courageous in bringing into this world a large number of children, are to be especially commended. You know of course historically, through the past 30-40 years, large Catholic families were pretty common. It doesn't seem to be quite as common today. I grew up in a family of 5 children, which I guess today, would be considered to be a large family. To be quite honest with you, when my sister Anne and David, my brother, came along I would occasionally complain to my parents and say, "Why did you have to have so many children?" Because we were poor; we didn't have very much money or anything. Why did we have to have so many children? From a selfish perspective, I thought we would have been much better off if we had fewer kids, so we could have nicer things, like a new car or a color TV, or whatever. Well, looking at it 20-30 years later, I realize that it was a blessing growing up with such a family, a large family of 5 children. Because ultimately, of course, the people you can depend upon in life are your family members. What a blessing it is for me to have three sisters and a brother that I can, to a certain degree, share my life with! What a blessing that is, to grow up in a large family! The Church is telling us that married couples that are courageous and generous bringing into life a large family are to be commended.

But you did notice in those sentences the words spoken by the Church, which say that this should be done after *prudent reflection and common decision*? In other words, the decision is made by the husband and wife. Earlier on, the Church teaches that it is the married couple themselves who must in the last analysis arrive at these judgments before God. It is the husband and wife before God, together who must make the decision about how wholly they are going to cooperate with God about bringing life into this world. I, as a priest, or any priest, or bishop, or even the Pope, cannot tell you, that you must have 5 children. No, it is your decision, husband and wife, before God, in consultation with God, in prayer before God, asking him, "Lord how many children do you want me to bring into this world?" That is the first thing to keep in mind. It is the common decision of the husband and wife before God. Also the Church says after prudent reflection, certain factors must be taken into consideration in coming to this decision. Some of those factors are listed as well by the Church. It involves the consideration of their own good and the good of their children already born or yet to come, the ability to read the signs of the times and their own situation on the material and spiritual level, and finally the estimation of the good of the family and society and of the Church. In other words the couple in making this decision before God in prayer should keep special factors in mind in coming to the decision.

There are several legitimate reasons for putting off having children or coming to an end to bringing children into this world. What are those legitimate reasons? Well, there are three possibilities. The first is this—we could call it financial: if a married couple is in a situation where they have no money, or no home, they may be wise and prudent in putting off having children. I know an example of a married couple who decided to put off having children for a year and-a-half. The reason they did so, is because the husband, at the time, was not making any money. He was doing an internship and the only person making any money in the family was the wife. So it was prudent of them to put off having children until the husband would begin a job in which he was making money. So there is the financial reason. The second reason for putting off having children would be the reason of genetics. In other words, if it was a pretty certain fact that a child to be born would be born with a serious birth defect, not a hangnail, but something serious, this could be a legitimate reason for putting off having children. Then finally, there would be a third reason, which is health. If it has been, once again, pretty certainly determined that a woman's health would be in danger by having another child, this could also be a legitimate reason for putting off having children, or having no more children in that person's lifetime. These are obviously serious reasons.

A couple must always keep in mind what the Church teaches as well, that married people should realize that in their behavior, they must not simply follow their own fancy. They must be ruled by conscience and conscience must be formed to the law of God, in the light of the teaching authority of the Church, which is the authentic interpreter of the Divine Law. So in coming to this decision, as husband and wife, before God, the couple must keep in mind the teaching of the Church. The Church is the interpreter of God's law. I am afraid today, that there are many married couples inside the Church who have forgotten that part. In making this decision to be open about human life, you must keep in mind the teaching of God's Church. The failure to do so, of course, is the failure to hear the Voice of God.

Now what is the advantage, then, of doing all this? The final sentence from *Gaudium et Spes*: "Whenever Christian spouses in a spirit of sacrifice and trust in Divine Providence carry out their duties of procreation with generous human and Christian responsibility, they glorify the Creator and perfect themselves in Christ." You become holy and closer to being a saint, when you fulfill these responsibilities in a spirit of sacrifice and trust in Divine Providence. Now, brothers and sisters, that leaves ultimately this question: If we are to be, as a married couple, generous in bringing human life into the world, and if there are certain circumstances in which we legitimately are able to put off having children what is the appropriate means? What is the legitimate and moral means with which we are to do that? Once again, that will be answered in the next homily.

Reprinted with permission, Godsplanforlife.com

The Church's Moral Teaching on Contraception, Part 3
By Father Anthony Kopp, O Praem

This is the third homily of a three-part series given by Fr. Anthony Kopp, O Praem, recorded at St. Kilian Church, Mission Viejo, CA.

My brothers and sisters, you may recall 2 weeks ago where we left off in our little series here on the issue of contraception. Today will be the third and final part of that series, and it is appropriate because today is "Respect Life" Sunday. As I am going to point out at the end of today's homily, it is appropriate because this issue is very much tied in with our modern day problem with respect, or lack thereof, for human life. The last time I left you with this question: "If a couple, before God, decides that it is appropriate to put off having children, what is the moral means, the good means for doing so?" How does a Catholic couple do that? The *Catechism of the Catholic Church* teaches us exactly how to go about doing so. In paragraph 2370 of the Catechism you read this: "Periodic continence, that is, the methods of birth regulation based on self-observation and the use of infertile periods is in conformity with the objective criteria of morality." The Catholic Church teaches us, and has always taught us, that the Catholic couple is to practice Natural Family Planning, the natural means, respecting God's order of things for spacing children. This is what the Church teaches us, in other words, to practice in marriage periodic abstinence or continence. Now that is not some new idea, something the Church just came up with recently that is arbitrarily imposed on married couples today. It is something you find in Sacred Scriptures. If you read the Book of Leviticus, chapter 15, it was commanded by God, in the Old Testament, for married couples to practice periodic abstinence.

Also, St. Paul in the first letter to the Corinthians says that a married couple should practice abstinence from time to time for the purpose of strengthening their prayer life. They should go apart for a time, strengthen that life, and then come back together. Now, what is the value of practicing Natural Family Planning? Well, the Catechism, in the next sentence, mentions several values. The first value is that these methods respect the bodies of the spouses, encourage tenderness between them, and favor the education of an authentic freedom. Now, I have talked to several married couples, both in my own family and outside of my own family. I have come up with a list of benefits, which they have related to me.

First of all, and I think most importantly, the practice of Natural Family Planning increases the amount, if you want to put it in those terms, of sacrificial love between the couple. Obviously if you are going to practice this method of Natural Family Planning, it requires sacrifice on the part of the couple. That sacrifice will be a result of, and will strengthen, the love found in that couple. Secondly, it strengthens or deepens the level of communication between the couple. Obviously, affection must be expressed in different ways. A couple practicing Natural Family Planning learn to do that. Finally, couples have noted to me, and this goes along with the idea of an increase of sacrificial love, that the practice of this method roots out, or tends to destroy selfishness (self-centeredness) in the marriage. If you have to sacrifice yourself for the good of your spouse when practicing this method, it helps you become less selfish.

We see at the societal level that this is the case. Studies have shown that for couples who practice Natural Family Planning, the divorce rate is less than 3%. Now my brothers and sisters, what is the divorce rate at the societal level, our society, which heavily promotes the use of contraception? It is over 50%! I can't help but wonder if we Catholics aren't on to something, that there isn't a great blessing in using this particular method. Now, in contrast, the Church has the following to say about contraception. In contrast, "every action, which whether in anticipation of the conjugal act, or in its accomplishment or in the development of its natural consequences, proposes whether as an end or as a means to render procreation impossible, is intrinsically evil." In other words, such acts are evil in themselves. So what's the Church talking about here? Well, the Church is talking about artificial contraceptives, sterilization, and of course, abortion. All of these things are intrinsic evils.

Another thing that is really important to know, my brothers and sisters, is that many of the contraceptives that are on the market today have tremendous side effects. When I first came into possession of the instruction sheet that goes along with the use of the Pill, I opened it and first of all, it's huge! And secondly, I was struck by the fact there was a whole column there that had possible side effects that a woman could endure by taking the Pill. I was thinking to myself, that if I was a husband and I loved my wife, would I want her to take anything like that, which could cause possible damage to her? Is that love, to put your spouse at risk like that in using such devices? I don't think so. Another thing we need to keep in mind with regard to contraceptives is that there are evil side effects. Many things about contraceptives today are not talked about. Many of these contraceptives today are abortifacients—they cause abortions. Women are often not aware of this fact. Many contraceptives fail to prevent conception, in which case they prevent the embryo from growing inside the woman's body. Abortion is caused after conception, and the woman is not aware of that fact.

You know, statistics in our country say that there are 1.4 million abortions a year. Well, the number is actually greater than that, hugely greater than that, because of all the abortions that are caused by abortifacient contraceptives. Now, when this is presented to people, namely that we are to use Natural Family Planning, and to shun contraceptives because they are intrinsically evil, or morally evil, right away people will say, "What's the difference? After all, the goal is the same—to put off having children. What's the difference?" Well, in answering that question, we need to keep in mind this: that the ends do not justify the means. That is a fundamental tenet of moral theology.

St. Paul also teaches that in his letter to the Romans. Just because I have a good end, doesn't mean that I can use any means to achieve it. Let's use a little example here. Yesterday, the football team of my school traveled to another school to play football. The other school was apparently much faster than we were, and so by half time we were down 28-7. Our coach could have said to our guys at half time, "Well, the goal is of course to win this game. Now, how are we going to do it? Well, we could, on the one hand, after half time, go and play our hardest. Or, we could, in the second half, injure the other team's players. That is a different means. We could, for example, get out our little files and sharpen our helmet buckles till they become razor sharp so the other team's players would be injured when we hit them." Now, that is pretty extreme. That did happen, by the way, last year in a football game in Texas. That's a different means. We see that those means are not equal. The end is the same. It is good to win the football game, but the means are not the same. One means is good, which is playing harder, which our guys did. We didn't win, but we came closer. Or, one uses the means of trying to injure the other team. That's evil. And that's the difference.

One means, Natural Family Planning, respects God's Order of things, respects the fertility and infertility of the married couple, has respect for the nature of the marital or conjugal act, which is good. Contraception does not. Contraception attempts to divide what God has joined together, namely the unitive aspect of marriage and the procreative aspect of the marital act. Those two are to be together, as our Holy Father himself in his encyclical, *Familiaris Consortio*, points out. He says this: "Thus the innate language that expresses the total reciprocal self-giving of husband and wife is overlaid through contraception by an objectively contradictory language, namely that of not giving oneself totally to the other. This leads not only to a positive refusal to be open to life, but also to a falsification of the inner truth of conjugal love, which is called upon to give itself a personal totality." In other words, the Holy Father is saying that by practicing contraception in marriage, the married couple is saying to each other, "You know I'm not really giving myself totally to you in this particular marital act."

Now when I first began this series about 4 or 5 weeks ago, I said that in my opinion, there is no greater evil in our society today, or in our Church, than the widespread use of contraceptives. Now why did I make this statement? Well, I could talk about this subject for hours. You probably don't want me to, so I am going to give a couple of illustrations. First of all, we see that contraceptives, or widespread use of contraception, leads to abortion. There is no question about that. We see that in every nation in the Western World, where contraception has been introduced, abortion has quickly followed. The same is true in the United States. In 1965, our Supreme Court in the case Griswold v. Connecticut, struck down all remaining laws on the books against the sale, possession and use of contraceptives. In that case, the basis for making the decision was the Supreme Court's finding in the Bill of Rights, of the so-called "right to privacy." Now where have we heard that before? Well, that language was used again in 1973 in Roe v. Wade. The so-called "right to privacy" which is no where found in our Constitution or in the Bill of Rights, but was invented by the Supreme Court to open the door to the use of contraceptives, then to abortion. Obviously, the use of contraception separates the marital act from its true end, namely procreation. When that happens, of course, the marital act becomes open to the use of anything that the parties involved want it to be used for. If then, the marital act is separated from procreation, what happens when procreation happens anyway? In that case, abortion is needed to eliminate the consequences. That is exactly what has happened in our society.

Secondly, contraception is a great evil because it has definitely weakened the Catholic Church in the United States. It has resulted in the breakdown of *authority*. Now this is very important because the Catholic faith is based on authority. First and foremost it is based on the authority of God's Word. We receive God's Word and must accept it and live according to it. To reject it is to make oneself no longer a follower of Jesus Christ. Our faith is based on the authority of God's Word. Secondly, it is based on the authority of Christ's Church that faithfully transmits and interprets for us God's word. To reject the authority of the Church is to reject the authority of Christ. It was in 1968, as I mentioned before, that the rejection of *Humanae Vitae* (which reiterated the Church's perpetual teaching on the issue of contraception) marked the first time many Catholics began to reject the teaching authority of the Church, thus rejecting the teaching authority of Christ. Obviously this has greatly weakened the Church. To no longer accept the authority of the Church is to no longer accept the authority of God.

What other evils have we seen since 1968? Well, I can't help but notice that Sunday Mass attendance has plummeted to a fraction of what it was just forty years ago. Well, obviously, if the Church doesn't have the authority to teach me in the area of contraception, then the Church doesn't have the authority to teach me to go to Mass on Sunday. I am free to choose whether to go or not. Many people have made that choice. I have also noticed, as a priest, that there has been a tremendous, even more significant than reduced Mass attendance, plummeting in the use of the Sacrament of Reconciliation. Once again that follows. If the Church doesn't have the authority to teach me in one area, then the Church can't tell me I need a priest to go to Confession. I can go to God; I am autonomous now and I make my own decision. I can go to God directly to have my sins forgiven. And, after all, if we are a married couple, using contraception, why would we go to Confession? I would be admitting that I am doing something that is contrary to the teaching of the Church, that the Church considers wrong. Why would I go to Confession and confess my sins? For many other moral issues as well, on which the Church teaches, we have seen the erosion of obedience. If the Church doesn't have the authority to teach me in one area, why should I follow the teaching in any area? Why can't I just decide for myself about anything that the Church might want to teach me?

Finally, I notice as a priest and an educator, that contraception is the root of why so many young people know so very little about our Catholic faith. The faith is not being passed on. Because, after all, once again, if you're a contracepting married couple, why would you teach your children the fullness of the Catholic faith, which is based on the authority of the Church that teaches us. Why would you do it? I am afraid that maybe with some religious educators teaching in our schools and religious education programs, the same thing is happening. Why would you teach the fullness of the Catholic faith if you don't accept it yourself? That's why I am afraid that in many programs, faith has been watered down. Fullness is not given. Because maybe they are embarrassed about the fullness of that faith and therefore a lot of times, sadly, they are occupied with doing art projects and the like while the fullness of the faith is not being passed on.

So, my brothers and sisters, as we come to the conclusion of all this, I think we really need in our society, especially in our Church, repentance, a change of heart. We desperately need that, a change of heart on this most important moral issue. All throughout the Old Testament God tells us that blessings will be bestowed upon those who follow God's law. That's so obvious in this issue. With the married couples that I've talked to who practice Natural Family Planning and respect the teaching of the Church, there are blessings, great blessings. On the other hand, God warns us in the Old Testament frequently, that to disobey His law is to draw upon ourselves curses. We see that in our society today. So my brothers and sisters, as Catholics, as leaven in the dough, we need a change of heart, repentance in this area. We would do well to heed the words of our Lord at the end of today's Gospel. It's a warning for us, if we don't change our hearts and our minds, on this issue. He says, "Therefore I say to you the kingdom of God will be taken away from you and given to a people that will produce His fruits."

May that not happen to us because of our resistance to God's word, to God's will in this area. My brothers and sisters, let us pray for a change of heart for Catholics in our world, a change of heart on this issue, a sense of repentance and openness to God's word, so that we might draw down upon us once again as a nation and as a Church, the blessings of God.

Reprinted with permission, Godsplanforlife.com. This three-part series is also available on CD. Contact God's Plan for Life at bgmurphy@cox.net or (949) 635-0019.

Anti-life Message Finds a Home in Contraception

By Most Reverend Paul S. Loverde, DD, STL, JCL
Bishop of Arlington, Virginia

"John is his name!" (Lk 1:63). These words of Zechariah, announced a few minutes ago in the gospel, identify for us the very special solemnity that we celebrate today, the birthday of Saint John the Baptist. There are only three times in the Church calendar that we celebrate the births of holy people: Christmas, the birth of Christ; September 8, the birth of the Blessed Mother; and today, the birth of John the Baptist. For the remainder of the "festival of saints," we celebrate their entrance into heaven, their birth into eternal life.

How appropriate it is for us today to also celebrate the Holy Sacrifice of the Mass, asking that all abortions cease and be no more. For John the Baptist brought a message of life into the world. We read in the responsorial Psalm, "I praise you for I am wonderfully made" (Ps 139:14a). In the *Catechism of the Catholic Church* we read about how we were "wonderfully made": "'Being man' or 'being woman' is a reality which is good and willed by God: man and woman possess an inalienable dignity which comes to them immediately from God their Creator (cf. Gen 2:7,22). Man and woman are both with one and the same dignity 'in the image of God.' In their 'being-man' and 'being-woman,' they reflect the Creator's wisdom and goodness'" (CCC 369). The prophet Isaiah, in the first reading, speaks of the Lord "who formed me as his servant from the womb" (Is 49:5).

Life is always created by God, not by man. Thus, it cannot be destroyed by man. Although a human person cannot fully reflect the complete glory of God, people can reveal part of that glory when they behave as images of God. We are made in God's image; we are to reflect God to others. How can we best image God? We can love as God loves. St. Cyprian said it another way, "When we call God our Father we ought also to act like sons…We should live like the temples of God we are, so that it can be seen that God lives in us" (*Office of Readings; Tuesday, 11th Week of Ordinary Time*).

Abortion results from a failure to love as Christ loves. Abortion has taken a traumatic toll on the lives of so many in this country because of a misconstrued idea of love, a self-gratifying love born out of selfishness, and not a sacrificial love, born out of complete self-donation. Additionally, often we hear that by using proper contraception, one can avoid pregnancy and thus reduce the number of abortions in our country. Our Holy Father speaks of the fallacy of this argument in the *Gospel of Life*. He says, "The Catholic Church is…accused of actually promoting abortion, because she obstinately continues to teach the moral unlawfulness of contraception." When looked at carefully, "This objection is clearly unfounded." "Certainly," he goes on to say, "from the moral point of view contraception and abortion are *specifically different* evils: the former contradicts the full truth of the sexual act as the proper expression of conjugal love, while the latter destroys the life of a human being; the former is opposed to the virtue of chastity in marriage, the latter is opposed to the virtue of justice and directly violates the divine commandment, 'You shall not kill.' But despite their differences of nature and moral gravity, contraception and abortion are often closely connected as fruits of the same tree" (13).

The contraceptive behavior, whereby one portrays a false love without being open to life, is inherently flawed. This anti-life attitude, which was fostered by Margaret Sanger when she founded the National Birth Control League (the predecessor of Planned Parenthood)[48] around 1914, promoted the belief that unlimited sexual pleasure without regarding whom the partner is or without worrying about bringing children into the world would "build marital happiness and stability."[49] Oh how that logic is flawed. Look at the divorce statistics in our country today! Look at the rise in child abuse, and in spousal abuse. "Woman and child abuse has multiplied 14 times since abortion became legal."[50] Yes, the anti-life message does not find its home only with abortion, but also with a contraceptive behavior, for as the Holy Father says in the *Gospel of Life*, they are "fruits of the same tree" (13). This anti-child attitude which draws people toward using contraceptives or abortifacients to prevent children, is the same attitude which leads to abortion when the methods fail.

But how does one act in a moral way in today's society? Let me offer some basic suggestions:

(1) The marital act has always been just that, reserved for the state of matrimony. The marital act outside of marriage "destroys the very idea of the family; [and] weakens the sense of fidelity" (CCC 2390). The marital act must be reserved for marriage.

---

[48] Kippley, *Sex and the Marriage Covenant*, 226.
[49] Ibid., 277.
[50] Nykiel, *No One Told Me I Could Cry*, 14.

(2) Children are a basic gift of marriage to be welcomed, not to be protected against. When a couple has "just reasons" to postpone the births of children, they should not come together during the fertile time. Thus, the couple manifests the true meaning of love, the giving of oneself for the good of the other, by practicing "the virtue of married chastity…with sincerity of heart" (CCC 2368).

(3) Married and engaged couples should learn the fertility awareness found in Natural Family Planning so that they make decisions on family size based upon knowledge of the wife's fertility and their own ability to be responsible parents for all of their children. Natural Family Planning classes are taught throughout the diocese, including here at Blessed Sacrament Parish.

Today we celebrate the Birth of Saint John the Baptist. As we continue the Eucharistic Sacrifice, let us be reminded also of the Baptist's death—a death which came about due to his defense of marriage. "Recall that Herod had had John arrested, put in chains, and imprisoned on account of Herodias, the wife of his brother Philip. That was because John had told him, 'It is not right for you to live with her'" (Mt 14:3-4). We all know the rest of the story of how Herodias' daughter was granted her wish from Herod to have the head of John the Baptist on a platter (Mt 14:6-11).

John the Baptist's life and death are centered on the celebration of life itself. As a prophet, he made clear the path for the Lord, announcing the Good News of salvation–our salvation—our life after death—in the person of Christ Jesus. As the Opening Prayer puts it, he was raised up "to prepare a perfect people for Christ the Lord." In his death, he continued to show the way to eternal life by teaching moral right and wrong in marriage.

So let us learn from the experience of St. John. Let us proclaim the Good News of the Gospel when it's easy and when it's difficult; when it is politically correct and when it is not; in season and out of season (2 Tim 34:1). May the courage of St. John the Baptist be with us as we continue to preach and to live the Gospel of Life!

Love Means Giving Oneself Away

By Most Reverend Thomas J. Olmsted
Bishop of Wichita, Kansas

20 January 2001

God created us in love; God created us out of love; God created us for love. God gave us two great commandments: "You shall love your God with all your mind, with all your heart, with all your strength and with all your soul. You shall love your neighbor as yourself." Love, then, is our origin, our destiny, our calling. If I do not love, if I do not experience love, my life remains an enigma to me and empty of meaning. Love alone makes life worthwhile.

That is why St. Paul writes: "If I speak in human and angelic tongues but do not have love, I am a resounding gong or a clashing cymbal. And if I have the gift of prophecy and comprehend all mysteries and all knowledge; If I have all faith so as to move mountains, but do not have love, I am nothing. If I give away everything I own, and I hand my body over so that I may boast but do not have love, I gain nothing" (1 Cor 13:1-3).

Thus, when we think of human dignity and the right to life of every human person, we begin by thinking of love. When we remember with sadness and abhorrence the infamous U.S. Supreme Court decision *Roe v. Wade,* which occurred 28 years ago, and when we try to understand our responsibility as individuals and as followers of Jesus for overturning that calamitous legal decision, we begin by focusing our attention on love. For love is our origin and our calling, our destiny and our hope. And while everything else in this world may pass away, love will not. Love, while tender; is strong. Love never fails (1 Cor 13:4-13).

But what is love? What does love look like? What is the difference between authentic love and its counterfeit? Fundamentally, we learn what love is from God, from the love of the three Persons of the Blessed Trinity; namely that love entails the giving and receiving of persons. "God so loved the world that he gave His only begotten Son." To love is to make oneself a gift for others and to receive others as a gift.

This is what *Christmas* is all about: God gave Himself to us. He made Himself a gift to us in the most human of terms. "The Word became flesh." He became a tiny child in the womb of the Virgin Mary.

This is what *Good Friday* is all about: God gave Himself to us, as an innocent victim on the Cross. He died so that we might live. He gave Himself over to death so that we might be saved from death.

This is what the *Last Supper* is about: God made Himself a gift for us, under the forms of bread and wine. Jesus took bread, broke it, and gave it to His disciples, saying: "This is my Body." Some of you in the pro-life movement may be familiar with Fr. Frank Pavone, founder of a movement called Priests for Life. In a recent article, he asked the question: "Did you ever realize that the same four words that were used by the Lord Jesus to save the world are also used by some to promote abortion? 'This is my body.' The same simple words are spoken from opposite ends of the universe, with meanings that are directly contrary to each other."

When Jesus spoke those words, He was pointing to Calvary, to what He would do with His body for the sake of others, how He would make His body a sacrifice so that we might have life. Moreover, He so completely makes Himself a gift for us that He invites us to share in His very life. He makes us members of His body, an awesome mystery of perfect love. Paradoxically, a person supporting abortion uses the same words to say the exact opposite: "This is my body. Don't tell me what to do with it! It's mine, and I can do whatever I want with it, even kill the life within it."

The same words can yield opposite results. Christ gives away His body so that we might have life and have it abundantly (cf. John 10:10). Abortion supporters hold tightly to their own bodies so that others might die. In giving His Body to us, Christ teaches the meaning of love: He says, "I sacrifice myself for the good of the other person." Abortion teaches the opposite of love: It says, "I sacrifice the other person for the good of myself" (Fr. Frank Pavone).

It is true for you and me to say, "This is my body," but why? Why is this body mine? Why did God give us that freedom and responsibility? So that we can do as Jesus did, so that we can obey Jesus' command at the Last Supper: "Do this in memory of me."

On the day you and I were born, our dad and mom said, "This is my body, given for you." They did not say, "This is my body, don't get in my way." This is the vocation and mission of parents. It is the way that we reverse *Roe v. Wade. A Culture of Life is built up one child at a time*, with men and women saying with Jesus, out of love for their spouse and out of love for each child God gives, "This is my body. As God has given my life to me, so I give it as a gift to you." Thus love consists in making oneself a gift for others.

There is one additional part of love, which follows naturally from its deepest meaning; namely, that love also means *gratefully receiving*. In fact, on the existential, human level, this is the most affirming part of love. This is what the Virgin Mary did, when she said to God, "Fiat, let it be done to me according to your word." She gratefully received into her body the gift of God's self; the Son of God became the son of Mary.

This is what Zechariah and Elizabeth did for John the Baptist; they gratefully received him as a gift from God. This is what husbands and wives do for each other, and why marriage is a sign of the love of Christ for His Church. This is what parents do for their children. Even prior to making their bodies a gift for their children, they receive with joy the gift of a child that comes from God.

Abortion is refusing to receive the child within as a gift. Not only is it not grateful for the gift of another human person, but abortion distorts the truth of the whole matter. Language gets twisted around; responsibility for others gets cast aside. Instead of being called a child, the unborn is called an aggressor or mere human tissue or some other such dehumanizing term. The refusal to see other persons as gifts of God, the choice to see them as unwanted burdens or intruders into privacy, is clear evidence of a Culture of Death.

Contraception follows this same false logic. For it refuses to receive one's spouse as a gift in his or her whole self. It says, "I will only receive you if you are not fertile." Not infrequently, it is said that there would be very few abortions if contraceptives were made easily available to all. Quite the opposite has proven to be true. In country after country, abortion only becomes widespread shortly after contraceptives are introduced into society. What follows legalized contraception is the development of a contraceptive mentality in which children are regarded as an obstacle to personal fulfillment. Any life that results from a sexual encounter which was supposed to be guarded from fertility by the Pill or other means thus becomes an enemy to be avoided at all costs. Abortion becomes the solution to failed contraception.

It is the love of God for the world that gives us cause to rejoice, that undergirds our hope. It is this love of God that forms the foundation of the dignity of every human being. From the very moment of conception, we are, each and everyone, created by God in love, and we are redeemed by the sacrifice of His Son. To each of us He says, "This is my body, given for you."

Let us rejoice in the love of God that is stronger than sin and more powerful than death. The love of the living Christ will never fail. Heaven and earth will pass away. *Roe v. Wade* will pass away; it is just a matter of time. But love will never pass away. The victory of Christ's love has already begun. His mercy works through us to build a culture of life and a civilization of love.

Mass Commemorating the 30th Anniversary of Humanae Vitae

By Justin Cardinal Rigali, JCD, Archbishop Emeritus of Philadelphia

Sunday, June 28, 1998

Gratitude for Embracing and Living the Message of Humanae Vitae

I wish to begin my homily this afternoon by expressing a word of gratitude to each of you. I am grateful for your desire to gather in anticipation of the thirtieth anniversary, this July 25th, of Pope Paul VI's Letter *Humanae Vitae*. I thank you not only for commemorating this anniversary, but for your dedication in living the teaching of *Humanae Vitae* in your family life.

I am grateful to *the doctors* who against enormous pressure by many of their peers have been faithful in their medical practice to the Church's vision of marriage and family. I thank those of you who for many years have led the efforts within the Archdiocese to proclaim the truth of the vision of life and love presented in *Humanae Vitae* and who have made available to couples within the Archdiocese the practical instruction to assist them in living marital chastity.

Most of all, I am grateful to all you couples present today who have embraced the teaching of *Humanae Vitae* and have incorporated this teaching into your married life. I commend you for your courage and fidelity to the vision of Christian marriage as expressed in *Humanae Vitae*, despite all the efforts to make you succumb to what can be described as a "contraceptive mentality," which is so pervasive in our culture.

Discipleship Is Never Easy, Never without Costs

Our readings for today's Mass remind us that *it has never been easy to follow the Lord*. Jesus was very honest about the hardships that would be required of those who accepted His call to discipleship: 'The foxes have lairs, the birds of the sky have nests, but the Son of Man has nowhere to lay his head" (Mt 8:20).

The Gospel also illustrates *the temptation to delay the commitment to discipleship*. There seem always to be "good" reasons for delaying our acceptance of the call of Jesus to come and follow Him. It is never difficult to develop excuses why now is not an opportune moment to surrender ourselves completely to the challenge of Christian discipleship.

Certainly, in the current cultural climate a married couple is barraged with numerous "reasons" why not to accept the full teaching of the Church with all its practical implications regarding the meaning and purposes of Christian married love.

The Catechism's Reaffirmation of Humanae Vitae

An essential element of the Church's teaching pertains to *the fecundity of marriage*. The *Catechism of the Catholic Church*, drawing on the formulations within *Humanae Vitae*, expresses the Church's teaching in this fashion:

Fecundity is a gift, an *end of marriage*, for conjugal love naturally tends to be fruitful. A child does not come from outside as something added on to the mutual love of the spouses, but springs from the very heart of that mutual giving, as its fruit and fulfillment. So the Church, which is on the side of life teaches that each and every marriage act must remain open to the transmission of life. This particular doctrine, expounded on numerous occasions by the Magisterium, is based on the inseparable connection, established by God, which man on his own initiative may not break, between the unitive significance and the procreative significance which are both inherent to the marriage act" (2366).

The *Catechism* elaborates on the practical implications of this inseparable connection between the unitive and procreative dimension of the marital act in this fashion:

A particular aspect of this responsibility concerns the *regulation of births*. For just reasons, spouses may wish to space the births of their children. It is their duty to make certain that their desire is not motivated out of selfishness but is in conformity with generosity appropriate to responsible parenthood. Moreover, they should conform their behavior to the objective criteria of morality…" (2368).

The *Catechism* goes on to specify what conforms to this objective criteria of morality:

Periodic continence, that is, the methods of birth regulation based on self-observation and the use of infertile periods, is in conformity with the objective criteria of morality. These methods respect the bodies of the spouses, encourage tenderness between them, and favor the education of an authentic freedom. In contrast, every action which, whether in anticipation of the conjugal act, or its accomplishment, or in the development of its natural consequences, proposes, whether as an end or as a means, to render procreation impossible is intrinsically evil…" (2370).

The *Catechism of the Catholic Church* restates what was contained in *Humanae Vitae*. In fact, each of the citations from the *Catechism* that I have just read relies greatly on the formulations on these matters found in *Humanae Vitae*.

The Critics of Humanae Vitae Misread the Consequences of Contraception

Pope Paul VI anticipated that the teaching of *Humanae Vitae* would not be easily received. Pope Paul VI acknowledged that the Church is not surprised to be, like Jesus Himself, *a sign of contradiction*. Pope Paul VI concluded that the Church has no alternative but with humble firmness to teach faithfully the entire moral law of which she is neither the author nor arbiter.

At the time of the promulgation of *Humanae Vitae*, there was intense opposition to its message. Those who argued that the Church should change her teaching on artificial contraception claimed that the widespread use of artificial contraception would strengthen Christian marriages, eliminate the problem of teen pregnancy, and diminish the perceived need for abortion and thus dramatically reduce the number of abortions.

Paul VI, on the other hand, argued that some of *the consequences of artificial contraception* would be increased occurrences of "conjugal infidelity and a general lowering of morality." As the utilization of artificial contraception has become more and more prevalent in the United States, our divorce rate has soared. Teen pregnancy has reached what some have termed epidemic proportions. The efforts to legalize abortion intensified after the promulgation of *Humanae Vitae* and with its legalization the number of abortions has skyrocketed.

Pope Paul VI in *Humanae Vitae* cautioned that once artificial contraception gained popular acceptance some governments would begin to impose contraception on their people. President Clinton's visit to China serves to remind us of the coercive nature of China's population policy that not only imposes contraception but also abortion.

Disrupting "the Ecology of Human Sexuality" Leads to Enslavement, Not Freedom

Paul VI was able to see clearly that once the "ecology" of the marital act was disturbed there would inevitably be dire consequences for the individual as well as for society itself. Paul VI recognized the inherent dangers of upsetting the balance that God had created in linking the sexual expression of human love with the awesome power to participate in the creation of new human life. Once *the connection between the expression of love and the power to transmit life* was severed, the trivialization of human sexuality, the devaluation of marriage and the loss of respect for human life were inevitable.

The acceptance of artificial contraception was the foundation for what would be termed "the sexual revolution." This revolution claimed to liberate. Yet, the "freedom" it offered was not *true freedom anchored in truth*, but a "freedom," as Saint Paul describes in our second reading today, "*that gives free rein to the flesh*" (cf. Gal 5:13-25). This "freedom" is indeed no freedom at all, but a new enslavement to an old master—lust and its destructive and uncontrolled cravings. Those who have eyes that desire to see can recognize clearly the truth of Pope Paul VI's insights as expressed in *Humanae Vitae* as well as the wisdom of the ancient truths upon which they were based.

The Antidote to the Contraceptive Culture Is True Christian Marriages Lived with Joy

What is the faithful Christian to do in a world that in so many ways has embraced values directly contrary to the moral law and the Gospel of Jesus Christ? Like the instruction in today's Gospel given by Jesus to the disciples who wanted to call down fire to destroy the Samaritans because they did not welcome them, we know that Jesus does not want us to respond harshly and violently to a world that is often quite hostile to the Christian understanding of human sexuality, marriage, and family (cf. Lk 9:54).

Rather, Jesus calls us as a Church to do precisely what so many of you in this Church have been doing for many years, namely to give unequivocal witness to the truth by *joyfully and faithfully living the vision of Christian marriage and family* as articulated in *Humanae Vitae* and reiterated in the *Catechism*.

Pope Paul VI in *Humanae Vitae* acknowledged that it is to married couples that the Lord entrusts the task of showing others the holiness of "the law which unites the mutual love of husband and wife with their cooperation with the love of God, the Author of human life." The Pope noted that married couples "become apostles and guides to other married couples" inspiring one another to embrace fully *the challenge of Christian marriage with all its hopes, anxieties and joys.*

Gratitude for Celebrating Love and Life in Daily Family Life

I conclude where I began, by thanking you for your efforts to understand and accept in its fullness the Church's teaching on Christian married life. Thank you for your courage, your fidelity, your generosity, your joy as you follow the example of the selfless love of Jesus in living your marital commitments of love, in accepting the awesome gift and challenges of Christian parenthood, and in discovering together what a gift you give to each other.

Thank you not only for "celebrating love and life" today, but for "celebrating love and life" each and every day in the manner in which you engage in the struggles and joys of Christian marriage, of Christian parenting, of Christian family life.

In this Holy Sacrifice of the Mass, through Christ and in the Holy Spirit, together we give thanks to the Father for the strength and grace that He has already infused into your hearts. And may you continue to be strengthened by the words that Jesus spoke to those who believed in Him: "If you live according to my teaching, you are truly my disciples; then you will know the truth, and the truth will set you free…That is why, if the Son frees you, you will really be free" (Jn 8:31-32, 36). Amen.

Perceiving the Contraception Connection

By Father Raymond Suriani
Saint Pius X Church, Westerly, Rhode Island

This homily (slightly abridged) was given on January 17, 1999 at the Cathedral of SS. Peter and Paul, Providence, RI.

As he stood on one of the banks of the Jordan River that day, he was surrounded by many people: people from Jerusalem, people from the countryside of Judea, they came to him in huge numbers. Of course, that was not unusual. In fact, Scripture indicates that it was always that way for John the Baptist. He truly was a charismatic personality, a man who could draw a crowd and then hold them spellbound by his teaching and preaching because he spoke the truth with such clarity and conviction. We're told that even some of those who hated him, like King Herod, were "captivated by his words."

So there he is, in the midst of this vast sea of humanity, ministering as he always did to hundreds of hungry souls, and he suddenly catches sight of someone coming toward him. Now please keep in mind that everyone else who was there that day saw this same individual making his way toward John. But to them, he was simply a young Galilean man, about 30 years of age; if they knew his family they would have said, "Oh yes, that's the son of Joseph, the carpenter from Nazareth."

In other words, when these hundreds of people looked at Jesus, they saw someone who appeared to be just like everybody else. But not John! John looked up, saw his cousin walking in his direction, raised his finger and said, "Look there! The Lamb of God who takes away the sin of the world." John the Baptist perceived what everyone else missed. And that's my point: John the Baptist perceived the deeper reality that everyone else missed.

My brothers and sisters, we live in a world right now in which a similar phenomenon is taking place with respect to the human person and basic life issues. For example, when we, as Christians, look at another human being, we see an individual of infinite value, an individual made in God's image and likeness, an individual with an immortal soul, an individual deserving of the utmost respect from the moment of conception to the moment of natural death.

But the sad and tragic fact is that many others do not *see* any of those things when they look at a fellow human being. When they look at another man or woman what they see is a cluster of cells, a product of conception, a disposable item, an object to be used for their own pleasure, a being no more valuable than a mosquito. They are like the crowds that stood with John that day on the banks of the Jordan River: they do not perceive the deeper reality of each person's dignity.

But unfortunately, the "perception problem," as I would call it, goes beyond this, even affecting some who would call themselves "pro-life." Here I'm thinking of those who do not perceive that abortion is the key social issue of our time. These people would say, "Of course I'm pro-life, but I think there are other social issues which are just as important as abortion: poverty, racism, violence, capital punishment and the like. Therefore all issues should be treated equally." The problem with that position is that it's contrary to what our Holy Father has said, and it's contrary to common sense.

As John Paul II told us during his pastoral visit of 1987:

"Feeding the poor and welcoming refugees, reinforcing the social fabric of this nation, promoting the true advancement of women, securing the rights of minorities, pursuing disarmament, while guaranteeing legitimate defense: all this will succeed *only if respect for life and its protection by law is granted to every human being from conception until natural death.* Every human person, no matter how vulnerable or helpless, no matter how young or how old, no matter how healthy, handicapped, or sick, no matter how useful or productive for society, is a being of inestimable worth created in the image and likeness of God. This is the dignity of America, the reason she exists, the condition of her survival, the ultimate test of her greatness: to respect every human person, especially the weakest and most defenseless ones, those as yet unborn."

The Holy Father, who certainly has the perception of John the Baptist, rightly understands that a person's position on the issue of abortion will ultimately affect his or her position on every other social and moral issue. Common sense should tell us that if we do not have respect for the innocent human life inside the womb, sooner or later we will not have any respect for the not-so-innocent human life outside the womb. We wonder why so many young people today exhibit such violent behavior. I'm convinced it's because they have grown up in a world where violence toward pre-born babies is considered acceptable behavior. And so these young people think to themselves: "If it's okay to kill that innocent baby, what is so bad about killing that guy in school who's been mean to me? He's certainly not innocent. If there are some innocent babies who don't deserve to live, then he certainly doesn't deserve to live."

Another area where the "perception problem" exists is what I would call "the contraception connection." This connection between contraception and abortion, as well as the connection between contraception and other social and moral evils, has been clearly affirmed by two great prophets of the latter 20th century: John Paul II and Paul VI. With the keen perception of John the Baptist, these two men have seen what so many intellectuals have completely missed.

In the *Gospel of Life*, our Holy Father says that although "they are specifically different evils" both abortion and contraception are "fruits of the same tree," rooted in "a self-centered concept of freedom" (13) Marvelously put! In other words, at the root of both abortion and contraception is pure, unadulterated human selfishness. The person using contraception says to his or her spouse, "You exist for me. Your purpose is to give me pleasure—to satisfy my desires." The action itself proclaims that message. The advocate of abortion says, "Pregnancy is a disease and children are a nuisance. I should not have to be bothered dealing with either one."

And then in 1968, that much-persecuted prophet Paul VI clearly enunciated the perennial teaching of the Church—that there are two purposes of marital sex: to have children and to establish a loving union between the spouses. And he indicated that whenever these two purposes are separated through a contraceptive act, it actually harms the relationship between a husband and wife.

Back then of course, most people laughed at such an idea. They said, "Holy Father, you've got to be kidding. Don't you realize artificial birth control is a great blessing! It will make for stronger marriages. Couples won't have to worry about unwanted pregnancies anymore. It will lessen marital anxiety. It will make for happier relationships and stronger families."

The Pope said, "Don't be fooled!" He warned that if artificial contraception ever became accepted and wide-spread, there would be many negative consequences: he said that there would be more infidelity in marriages; he said that women would be treated more and more like objects by men; he said that morals would be lowered in society as a whole; and he predicted that some governments would try to push birth control on poor countries—just like the United States does today.

On every count, he was right! He had the perception of the Baptist when so many others were blinded by their hormones! Praise God, some 30 years later, many are now finally seeing the truth and embracing it—so there is hope!

On that note, I just finished reading a great book that I'll recommend to you. It's called *Physicians Healed*, and it's published by *One More Soul*. It consists of personal testimonies by 15 doctors (obstetricians, gynecologists, and family practitioners) who have stopped giving all contraception to their patients, and not all of them are Catholic! They have all become promoters and teachers of Natural Family Planning, which, contrary to popular belief, is *not* the old "Rhythm Method." It's a scientific method of fertility awareness which can be used either to achieve or avoid a pregnancy, and which, when used properly, is acceptable to the Church and is as effective as any means of contraception.

One of the doctors cited in this book wrote the following in his personal testimony. This, I would say, speaks volumes:

I now realize that contraception is neither good nor necessary. May the Lord forgive me for those human embryos I eliminated with IUDs. Mea culpa. May the Lord forgive me for those human embryos I eliminated with Norplant. Mea culpa. May the Lord forgive me for those human embryos I eliminated with the rape protocol. Mea culpa. May the Lord forgive me for those human embryos I eliminated with birth control pills. Mea maxima culpa.

As physicians, we should realize that the popes have far more wisdom on ethical issues than we could imagine. We can only appreciate their wisdom by following their teachings. We are not smart enough to overrule their infallible reasons. Eight years of medical training does not counterbalance 2,000 years of Catholic tradition. To learn, we must adopt an open-minded attitude of humility and obedience.

Now there's a doctor with the insight and perception of John the Baptist!

May all of us in this cathedral tonight be willing to open our minds to the fullness of God's truth as taught by his Church, so that we can become true apostles for life in this present culture of death. May we follow the example of John and proclaim this truth without compromise and without shame. And may we always point to Jesus like John did, telling those who have had abortions and performed abortions and used contraception, "Don't despair. Look, there is the Lamb of God, who will take away your sin—if you simply go to him in Confession;" and saying to the whole world, "Look, there is the Lamb of God who came to give us life—not death—*life*! Treasure this gift, nurture this gift on earth, and receive the fullness of the gift someday in heaven."

Amen.

"This Sort of Talk Is Hard to Endure! How Can Anyone Take It Seriously?"

By Father Joseph Taphorn
Archdiocese of Omaha, Nebraska

My brothers and sisters, today the Church concludes the section from the Gospel of John on the Bread of Life. We have heard for five weeks now about the necessity of receiving Jesus in the Eucharist. But the disciples are still protesting; their reaction, we must admit, seems perfectly logical. How can he possibly offer us His body to eat and His blood to drink? This type of talk is foolish, they say. We benefit from twenty centuries of belief in the Eucharist, so we may not share these same doubts, as did the disciples. But do we doubt other teachings of Christ and His Church? Do we find them hard to accept?

What about our second reading from Ephesians: *"Wives should be submissive to their husbands as if to the Lord because the husband is head of his wife just as Christ is head of His body, the Church, as well as its savior…Husbands, love your wives, as Christ loved the Church. He gave himself up for her to make her holy…Husbands should love their wives as they do their own bodies."*

How many young people today would be willing to choose this as a reading at their wedding? It is a tough teaching, and we may be tempted to say, like the disciple, "This is too much! This sort of talk is nonsense!"

In this passage, St. Paul eloquently presents the true meaning of Christian marriage. It is not something that we should turn off at the outset because we dislike words like "submissive." Rather, we should strive to understand and appropriate the full meaning of what God is showing us in this passage.

The model for Christian marriage that Paul presents is that of Christ and His Church. Christ gives himself up for His bride, the Church. He dies on the Cross, surrendering His life for those whom He loves. Husbands, like Christ, should give up their lives for their wives and children. They should be willing to die to themselves and their own desires in deference to the ones they love. This is why husbands are seen as the providers and guardians of the family. They are willing to die, if necessary, to save the lives of their loved ones.

The blockbuster movie, "Air Force One," starring Harrison Ford as the President of the United States, depicts the hijacking of Air Force One by communist terrorists. Along with his aides, the President's family is also aboard. The Secret Service rushes him to a special escape pod and insists that he flee to safety. That is his duty to his country, the prevailing logic goes. Unbeknownst to his aides, our hero climbs out of the escape pod before it ejects and remains on board the plane. He knows that he must protect and defend his family, even if it means sacrificing his own life. While this is not a recommendation for the movie, and the tale may seem fantastic, the point is well made. The love that the President shows for his wife and children is boundless; he would rather die than abandon his family. This is the love that Christ has for the Church, and it is the love that husbands should have for their wives.

In light of this, it is much easier to understand Paul's words that wives should be submissive to their husbands. Permit me to explain. In our reading Paul recalls the words of Genesis which speak of the creation of Adam and Eve: *"For this reason a man shall leave his father and mother, and shall cling to his wife, and the two shall be made into one."* The two become one; their identity is found in each other. It is for that reason that a couple's name changes after marriage. They are no longer two, but one. This week my parents will celebrate their 36th wedding anniversary. On that day 36 years ago they were no longer James Taphorn and Joan Schram, but Mr. and Mrs. James Taphorn. From this sign alone we can see that there should not be a clash of wills in a marriage, as if two single people were both trying to run the same household. No, a husband who loves his wife as Christ loves the Church would not demand anything inappropriate or selfish; and a wife who is submissive to her husband in the sense Paul describes here would be equally willing to make sacrifices for the sake of her spouse and children. What we are talking about here then is a *mutual submission, a mutual self-offering* of the two individuals for the sake of the one family. Yes, Christ and the Church are one just as husbands and wives are one. In both cases there is a love so intimate, so exclusive, and so faithful, that the identity of one is found in the other.

For married couples, the marital act is the sign of this exclusive and faithful love. Sex is not something bad or dirty; it is holy and sacred. And for this reason it is to be expressed only in the context of marital love, marital fidelity. Sex outside of marriage, outside of this total commitment and self-surrender cheapens a holy act and defiles it; it reduces sex to something less than it is.

Because the marital act is the sign of total self-surrender, it naturally bears fruit. It enhances the love couples share and is the instrument God has designed for the transmission of new life. You might say that the love a couple has for each other can be named—Mary, or Billy, or Johnny. It is for this reason that contraception is gravely wrong. It betrays the meaning of the marital act. It is no longer a *total* self-giving; it is saying, at the same time, "yes, but no."

Is this kind of talk too much to endure? Is Father crazy? Can he really mean what he is saying? Yes, I do. This is not an easy teaching. I know that. I remember when I was a junior in high school at Creighton Prep in Omaha. I took a moral values class. In class our teacher presented the Church's teaching on contraception. I thought it was crazy. It took me a long time to understand and accept what the Church teaches. It came about as the result of much prayer and study.

Jesus, too, knows that this is not an easy teaching. And if you find yourself struggling with this, you are not alone. But know that Jesus shares His life and His grace with us, and He is always calling us to give more and more of ourselves, so that we can receive more and more of His grace in our lives. Like many of the disciples, Peter probably did not fully understand the teaching on the Eucharist. But he knew Jesus, and was willing to trust Him. God gave him the grace to believe.

If you find this teaching hard to take, I invite you to be open to what the Church offers, to really learn what the Church teaches and why. She knows that couples may have a genuine need to plan their families and that right is to be respected. But there is a right way and a wrong way. Here in Norfolk we are blessed to have a Natural Family Planning center just a couple of blocks from here at the east campus of Faith Regional. Natural Family Planning is the *right* way. Please feel free to talk to me anytime about questions or struggles you might have with this teaching. No one condemns you. Rather, the words Jesus offers are spirit and life.

When we approach the altar today to receive the Eucharist, we are given an invitation and a challenge. Will we be like the disciples who broke away and left the company of Jesus and said, *"This sort of talk is hard to endure! How can anyone take it seriously?"* Or will we be like Peter and apostles, who trusted and said to Him, "Lord, to whom shall we go? You have the words of eternal life"?

Additional Resources

Learn more about the Church's teaching on the harm of contraception and the blessings of children with these resources, available from One More Soul....

Adam and Eve after the Pill

by Mary Eberstadt
Published by Ignatius Press

An incisive, lively and illuminating commentary on the effects of the Pill (and other means of intentional sterility) on our society and culture. This is a "must read" for those who want to know what has happened to our society and what to do about it.

The Art of Natural Family Planning Student Guide

Published by Couple to Couple League

This is the main resource book of the Couple to Couple League, which mainstreamed the Sympto-Thermal Method of Natural Family Planning. It is stuffed with helpful information including how to apply NFP and how to handle unusual NFP situations.

The Billings Method

by Dr. Evelyn Billings
Published by Billings Family Life Centre

Dr. Evelyn Billings, with her husband, John, refined the Ovulation Method now used all over the world. In this book she describes in detail how to use the Billings method and its scientific basis. Today there are over a million copies in print in 22 languages.

The NaProTechnology Revolution

by Thomas W. Hilgers, MD
Published by Beaufort Books, New York, New York

A comprehensive guide to the NaProTechnology system of Natural Family Planning and of treatment of various female reproductive diseases using NaProTechnology. A wide range of female reproductive diseases have been treated with amazing success by these methods.

Birth Control and Christian Discipleship

by John F. Kippley
Published by the Couple to Couple League

The author reviews how all Christian churches strongly condemned contraception up to 1930, but many began accepting it after that, leading to the disastrous sexual revolution. He points out that there is still a clear path for churches to reorient and reject this evil.

Breast Cancer, Its Link to Abortion and the Birth Control Pill

by Chris Kahlenborn, MD
Published by One More Soul

Based on six years of study and a meticulous analysis of hundreds of scientific papers and other sources, Dr. Chris Kahlenborn documents the effect that abortion and hormonal contraception have on breast cancer, as well as uterine, cervical, liver, and other cancers, and even the transmission of AIDS! Hormonal contraceptive use before first full term pregnancy is found to increase risk of breast cancer by at least 40%. The book gives special attention to black women, to various populations of the world, and to effective steps for prevention. This is a very timely and powerful work.

Catholics and Contraception

by Leslie Woodcock Tentler
Published by Cornell University Press

A detailed history of how the Catholics of the USA went, in a very short time, from almost complete rejection of contraception to almost complete acceptance of it. Tentler does an excellent job analyzing and presenting this history and ends with a strong plea for the US Catholic authorities to stand up to this disaster.

A Crash Course in the Theology of the Body (Naked Without Shame, second edition)

by Christopher West
Published by The Gift Foundation

This CD lecture series outlines John Paul II's Theology of the Body, a new synthesis that includes an extremely positive approach to Christian sexuality and also gives solutions to moral problems that have caused confusion for generations. Truly a wonderful and innovative presentation. A comprehensive study guide for this series is also available.

Discovering the Feminine Genius

by Katrina J. Zeno
Published by Pauline Press

The author explains how to be a woman in the most luminous terms, based on the theology of Pope John Paul II. Also very powerful for men.

God's Plan for a Joy-filled Marriage

by Christopher West
Published by Ascension Press

A complete set of tools for giving Marriage Preparation students what they need for a truly happy marriage. The set includes a set of lectures on CD and on DVD along with a Leader's Guide for the main presenter and a Student's Guide with all sorts of material to help the couples absorb the material.

Good News about Sex & Marriage

by Christopher West
Published by Servant Publications

Subtitled: "Answers to Your Honest Questions about Catholic Teaching," this book takes dozens of the toughest questions on human sexuality and brings them Christopher West's enthusiasm, great insight, and joy in the truth. In his hands the most vexing problems in the Catholic approach to sexual love definitely become Good News.

Heaven's Song, Sexual Love as It was Meant to Be

> by Christopher West
> Published by Ascension Press

> Within the Theology of the Body, John Paul II composed wonderful teachings on the Song of Songs and on the story of Sarah and Tobias from the book of Tobit. In this book, Christopher West takes these treasures and embeds them in stories of people he has known who received healing for their distorted sexual values through the Theology of the Body. This is the best book on sexuality I have ever read.

Humanae Vitae: A Challenge to Love

> by Pope Paul VI
> Published by New Hope Publications

> Professor Janet Smith here provides a new translation of *Humanae Vitae,* directly from the original Latin, and adds an article on themes and language of the encyclical. Many people consider this translation to be the most accurate and accessible available.

Into the Heart

> by Christopher West
> Published by Ascension Press

> A superb introduction to the Theology of the Body with several study aids: a set of lectures on CD and on DVD, a Leader's Guide for the instructor, and a Student's Guide for participants.

Love and Fertility

> by Mercedes Arzu Wilson
> Published by Family of the Americas Foundation

> An illustrated how-to manual of the Ovulation Method of fertility awareness, complete with charts and other helpful materials. The female fertility cycle is compared to the plant growth cycle, and simple, direct instructions are given for achieving or postponing pregnancy.

Love and Responsibility

by Karol Wojtyla
Published by Ignatius Press

Karol Wojtyla (later Pope John Paul II) applies personalist philosophy to human sexuality, love, and marriage. As Pope, he took this same body of thought and, starting with Scripture, built his magnificent Theology of the Body. This is a challenging book, but extremely rewarding.

Marriage Is for Keeps, Wedding Edition

by John F. Kippley
Published by Couple to Couple League

The ultimate marriage preparation book. Discusses the meaning of the marriage commitment, NFP, children, birth control, and many other important topics. Includes the complete Marriage Rite and Readings. The perfect engagement present.

New Perspectives on Contraception

by Donald DeMarco, PhD
Published by One More Soul

Examining contraception from several perspectives, Professor DeMarco illuminates how contraception separates people from their spouses, from God, and even from their own best interests. He probes the ideas of choice, personhood, suffering, reality, and love, with poignant and often humorous insights and a style that entertains and enlightens.

Physicians Healed

Edited by Cleta Hartman
Published by One More Soul

Moving stories of 15 physicians who do not prescribe contraceptives and who promote Natural Family Planning. These are powerful accounts of conversion, courage, and conviction. Learn what moved these doctors to risk losing patients, income, and the respect of their peers. John Cardinal O'Connor of New York stated: "It is indeed inspiring to read of the spiritual journeys of these faithful physicians, and especially of their honesty and perseverance." Share this with your physician; many have been converted.

Sterilization Reversal, A Generous Act of Love

    Edited by John L. Long
    Published by One More Soul

    Touching personal stories of 20 couples who chose sterilization as a solution for family difficulties and then were given the grace to choose healing and wholeness in a radical way. Appendices in the book cover medical aspects of reversing vasectomy and tubal ligation and pastoral reflections on sterilization and reversal by a bishop and a priest.

Why Humanae Vitae Was Right

    Edited by Janet E. Smith, PhD
    Published by Ignatius Press

    The editor gathers a stellar group of philosophers and theologians to comment on aspects of *Humanae Vitae*. The Church's teaching on contraception is superbly defended based on the Bible, Church teaching, and Natural Law. This book will make fascinating reading for the serious student.

One More Soul **offers a number of other books and audio/video resources. CDs can be purchased individually or in sets. OMS also offers an extensive selection of pamphlets, which can also be purchased individually or in bundles.**

For more information, see our catalogue at www.omsoul.com or call (800) 307-7685.

What is One More Soul?

One More Soul (OMS) is a non-profit organization dedicated to spreading the truth about the blessings of children and the harmful effects of contraception. We provide a wide variety of educational resources and services aimed at opening our culture to God's design for marital love.

We were founded in 1993 by Steve Koob and Mary Ann Walsh, two Dayton, Ohio, pro-life veterans. Through their pro-life work they realized that the foundation of abortion is contraception, and that contraception must be rooted out before abortion would be rejected by our culture. The more they learned about contraception, the more they were convinced that it was the root of abortion and numerous other social ills.

Steve and Mary Ann felt a responsibility to share what they had learned with their fellow pro-lifers, Christians, and the world. They decided that the most efficient way to do this was to distribute educational resources explaining the truth about contraception, and promoting a pro-child attitude. They founded ***One More Soul*** to accomplish their goals. The name "One More Soul" sprang from their hope that through the grace of God and their efforts "one more soul" would be created for the kingdom of God. Since the creation of a soul is more awesome than the creation of the whole material universe, one soul would more than justify any amount of effort.

About the Author

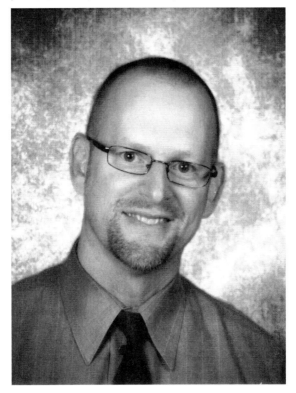

Jason T. Adams is the Headmaster at Lumen Christi Catholic School in Indianapolis, Indiana., where he resides with his wife, Linda, and their five children. Jason holds the degrees of Bachelor of Arts in Secondary Education, from Purdue University, and Master of Arts in Theology from the Franciscan University of Steubenville. He has written and spoken on Catholic faith, and a variety of pro-life, pro-family topics. He continues to consult on projects for One More Soul (this book's publisher).

Jason converted to Catholicism from evangelical Protestantism in 1993 after five years of inquiry, during which time he struggled with many doctrinal issues, including the issue of contraception. Jason and Linda have used Natural Family Planning to successfully postpone and achieve pregnancy throughout their marriage. Jason comments about his family: "All of our children have been blessings, but each in a different way. God is good."